THE SACRED CANOPY

THE SACRED CANOPY

Immersive Nature-Based Practices For Mind, Body, and Soul
195 experiences in 24 unique settings

iRewild Institute
Ocala, FL

Written by
Ida M. Covi

Cover Illustated by
Daniel Desembrana

Select illustrations within the book by
Daniel Desembrana

Additional clip art and watercolor compositions by
Julia Dreams and Zeppelin Graphics available through Envato

Edited by
Hannah Irish

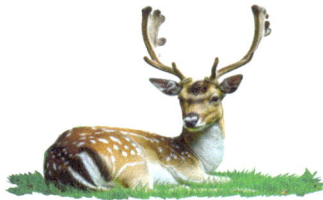

For our world . . .
a world in which we all belong

This is an iRewild Institute Book

Ocala, Florida

www.iRewild.com

iRewild Institute is an international organization working to bring the human soul back into a deeper, more conscious relationship with nature. For information about how you may participate in its programs, please visit our website.

Written By Ida M. Covi

Illustrated by Daniel Desembrana

Edited by Hannah Irish

Published by

iRewild Institute, Ocala, FL, USA

ISBN: 979-8-218-48172-8

Library of Congress Cataloging in Publication Data

iRewild Institute

The Sacred Canopy

Immersive Nature-Based Practices For Mind, Body, and Soul

195 experiences in 24 unique settings

Disclaimer:

This book is intended for informational purposes only. The publisher and authors are not responsible for any adverse effects or consequences resulting from the use of any suggestions or procedures described within this book. All readers should consult with a qualified professional before attempting to implement any practices or recommendations contained herein.

With the deepest gratitude to Nature...

For it's in the hushed whispers of the forest and the gentle lapping of waves that we find the deepest realms of human existence. Nature is not just a place—it's the breath of our soul.

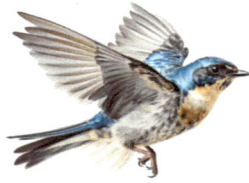

TABLE OF CONTENTS

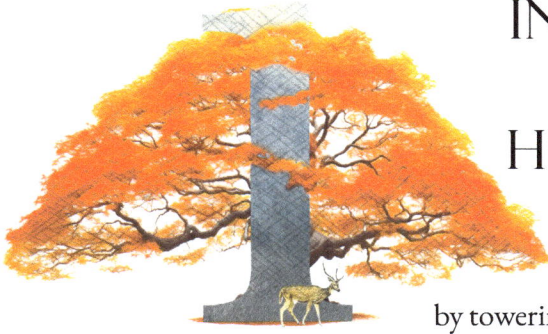

INTRODUCTION: NATURE'S HEALING TOUCH

Picture yourself in a serene forest, surrounded by towering trees, their leaves gently swaying in the breeze. Inhale the earthy scent of the forest floor and listen to the melodic symphony of bird songs above. Welcome to the world of nature therapy, where nature becomes your companion, offering healing and tranquility in the embrace of its green sanctuary. As we embark on this journey, I invite you to leave behind the hustle and bustle of everyday life and immerse yourself in the soothing embrace of nature. Together, we'll explore the profound tie between nature and wellbeing, discovering the hidden wonders and therapeutic benefits that only the natural world can offer. So, let's take a mindful step into the heart of nature and unlock the revitalizing secrets that await us.

It's fascinating how our minds are shaped by the fast-paced, tech-driven world we live in. But deep down, our bodies have this innate connection with nature. In recent years, researchers have delved deep into this, uncovering a wealth of health benefits tied to spending time in the natural world. It's not just about the beauty of nature; it's something our bodies truly need.

Spending time in forested areas for the purpose of enhancing health, wellbeing, and happiness has been practiced in Japan for several centuries, where it is now referred to as 'Shinrin-yoku' [sheen-din-yoock-ooo], which translates as "Forest Bath," a poetic name for: walking slowly through the woods or forest; inhaling the forest air while immersing yourself in the natural surroundings; mindfully using all your senses, opening them to the forest atmosphere; noticing body sensations while fostering an emotional connection to the landscape.[1] This particular kind of nature therapy has its origins in Buddhist nature-connection practices and the beliefs within the Shinto religion about the sacred healing powers of forests.[2]

---

1   Li, Qing. "Effects of forest environment (Shinrin-yoku/Forest bathing) on health promotion and disease prevention—the Establishment of 'Forest Medicine'—." Environmental Health and Preventive Medicine 27 (2022): 43. https://doi.org/10.1265/ehpm.22-00160.

2   Livni, Ephrat. "Japanese 'forest medicine' is the science of using nature to heal yourself—wherever you are." Quartz, February 21, 2018. https://qz.com/1208959/japanese-forest-medicine-is-the-art-of-using-nature-to-heal-your-self-wherever-you-are.

For the past forty-plus years, researchers around the world have been studying the benefits of nature, and specifically forests, on human health and wellbeing. These studies show that exposure to forests and trees can:[3]

> boost the immune system,
>
> lower blood pressure,
>
> reduce stress,
>
> improve mood,
>
> increase ability to focus, even in children with ADHD,
>
> accelerate recovery from surgery or illness,
>
> increase energy level,
>
> and improve sleep.

Japanese researchers have also been studying whether time in forests may even help prevent certain kinds of cancer. Forest bathing is included as part of Japan's healthcare system, with many companies subsidizing weekends for their employees to visit forests to reduce burnout in the workplace.

In essence, nature-based experiences, backed by science, are transformative and have the potential to foster a better quality of life. Are you wondering how much time in nature is necessary for people to feel healthier and more content? It might surprise you: just two hours a week is sufficient, and it doesn't have to be all at once.

The University of Exeter conducted a study involving 20,000 individuals.[4] Researchers discovered that individuals who dedicated two hours each week to being in green spaces, such as parks or natural environments, whether in a single visit or spaced out over several outings, were far more likely to report improved overall health and enhanced psychological wellbeing than those who don't. The crucial factor was the consistent two-hour duration. These strong and positive outcomes were consistent across various ethnic communities, occupations, income levels, illnesses, and disabilities. Other research has shown that inhaling forest aerosols during a walk boosts natural killer (NK) cells in the immune

---

3   Immerse Yourself In A Forest For Better Health." New York State Department of Environmental Conservation. Accessed July 20, 2024. https://dec.ny.gov/nature/forests-trees/immerse-yourself-for-better-health.

4   White, M.P., Alcock, I., Grellier, J. et al. "Spending at least 120 minutes a week in nature is associated with good health and wellbeing." Scientific Reports 9, 7730 (2019). https://doi.org/10.1038/s41598-019-44097-3.

system,[5] [6] enhancing the body's ability to combat tumors, infections, and other health challenges.

As human beings, the core of our very essence is intertwined with our physical existence. Our bodies—consisting of flesh, blood, bones, nerves, and the mind—serve as the channels through which we encounter both ourselves and the surrounding world.

In my role as an eco-psychologist, I strive to enrich our engagement with nature, endeavoring to cultivate an immersive, transformative, and deeply meaningful experience. This also addresses an additional dimension of nature's importance in the lives of many: its spiritual dimension.

Humanity has a deep desire to seek out and experience the sacred, the mystery in everyday life. The sacred often reveals itself through a deep reverence for nature as we recognize the interconnectedness between humans, the natural world, and the cosmos. People seek to understand the larger cosmic order and our place within it. In nature, we often recognize the presence of a sacred or a transcendent realm that influences and gives meaning to the physical world. In the presence of nature, we find ourselves in closer communion with a higher power, freely expressing our gratitude and joy, as well as our sorrows, with a deep sense of connection. Regardless of our individual religious affiliations or lack thereof, nature remains a universal force that embraces each and every one of us.

My role is to help you open a door, to slow down, both physically and mentally. Immersing ourselves in purposeful nature-connection practices or 'invitations' creates a soul-nourishing experience that may not only enhance your relationship with nature, but also boost the therapeutic and restorative effects of nature toward improving your health and wellbeing.

5   Li, Q., M. Kobayashi, Y. Wakayama, H. Inagaki, M. Katsumata, Y. Hirata, K. Hirata, et al. "Effect of Phytoncide from Trees on Human Natural Killer Cell Function." International Journal of Immunopathology and Pharmacology 22, no. 4 (2009): 951–59. https://doi.org/10.1177/039463200902200410.

6   Li, Qing. "From a Feeling to a Science." Essay. In Forest Bathing: How Trees Can Help You Find Health and Happiness, 57-116. New York, NY: Viking, 2018.

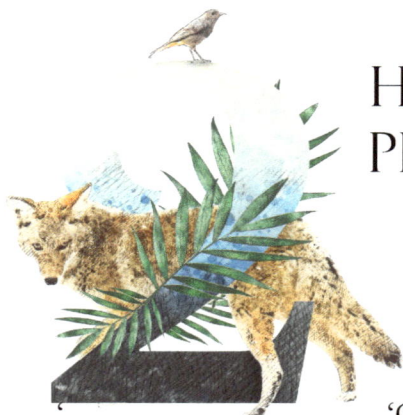

HOW DO NATURE-BASED PRACTICES DIFFER FROM JUST A WALK IN THE WOODS?

The primary differences are intention and distance covered. 'Ordinary' walks often have a geographical goal, such as getting to the top of a hill or mountain, or walking all the way around a lake. Quite often we can be so focused on getting to where we want to go that we fail to notice what is around us. On a nature therapy walk, the intention is to increase our awareness of our environment and increase our nature-connection. The goal is achieving a positive and beneficial state of mind, the experience of reduced stress, and increased relaxation, rather than reaching a destination or covering a particular distance. The urban century is upon us; it is estimated that two-thirds of the global population will reside in cities by 2050.[7] This expansion engulfs natural landscapes and distances people from their innate connection with nature. Under the momentum of modernization, people in most areas of the world typically spend 90% of their lives within some type of building.[8] Consequently, as we move into city living, and indoors, we undergo a dramatic disconnect from the natural world. Deprived of our experiences in nature, with less need and use of them, our senses become atrophied.[9]

Furthermore, overtime, life's pains and the overwhelming plights vying for our attention drive us to numb our senses, compounding the withdrawal of our attention from sensorial experience. This psychological phenomenon of psychic numbing causes us to feel indifferent to the plights and suffering of other people and of our planet.[10]

7　　Li, Qing. "Effects of forest environment (Shinrin-yoku/Forest bathing) on health promotion and disease prevention—the Establishment of 'Forest Medicine'—." Environmental Health and Preventive Medicine 27 (2022): 43. https://doi.org/10.1265/ehpm.22-00160.

8　　Evans, Gary W., and Janetta Mitchell Mccoy. "When Buildings Don't Work: The Role Of Architecture In Human Health." Journal of Environmental Psychology. 18, no. 1 (1998): 85–94. https://doi org/10.1006/jevp.1998.0089.

9　　Kesebir, Selin, and Pelin Kesebir. "How Modern Life Became Disconnected from Nature." Greater Good, September 20, 2017. https://greatergood.berkeley.edu/article/item/how_modern_life_became_disconnected_from_nature.

10　　Covi, Ida. Rewilding the Senses: Bringing the Human Soul Back Into Conscious Relationship with Nature, 3-5. Ocala, FL: iRewild Institute, 2020.

With each passing day, the relentless news stories detailing unending wars, social injustices, and the intensifying climate crisis, coupled with our own individual challenges, leave us feeling profoundly inundated, causing our sensory networks to tire, shut down, and become emotionally indifferent. Eventually, whether by choice or unconsciously, we build energetic walls around ourselves for protection. When this happens, we disconnect, distancing ourselves from our own nature and that of our natural world and its life-giving benefits. While temporary numbness can be beneficial and may serve a purpose, it becomes detrimental in the long run, depriving us from fully experiencing the deepest realms of human existence.

It's a systemic disconnect at a deep level, and, as science is discovering, there is a synergistic and inseparable relationship between planetary and personal wellbeing—the needs of the one are relevant and crucial to the needs of the other.[11] We forget that human beings also embody nature and belong to the wider natural world. Isolated from the world that enfolds us, we lose a vital source of our wellness. We fall short of experiencing the richness of our world, and at the same time we leave behind a natural world in crisis.

When we deprive our senses, we steal our own life experiences away from ourselves. We retain an unrealistic perspective about our lived reality. Knowing that we possess the abilities to self-evidence new experiences, to understand our sensory experiences, and examine our inner lives, leads us to gain further knowledge of what it is 'to exist' and to experience the deepest realms of human existence, a life filled with richer meaning and awe.

The idea of humans having five senses is rooted in ancient history. The Greek philosopher Aristotle (384-322 BCE) was the first to tell us that we perceive reality, that we collect and respond to information and sensations about our world, through our five senses: sight, hearing, touch, taste, and smell.[12] With advancements in science, scientists now count from twenty-two to as many as thirty-three sensory systems depending on the method of neurological classification.[13] We can sense direction, balance, body tempera-

11   Covi, Ida. Rewilding the Senses: Bringing the Human Soul Back Into Conscious Relationship with Nature, 4. Ocala, FL: iRewild Institute, 2020.

12   Aristotle. De Anima, Book II, c. 350 BCE.

13   Durie, Bruce. "Senses Special: Doors of Perception." New Scientist, January 26, 2005. https://www.newscientist.com/article/mg18524841-600-senses-special-doors-of-perception/.

ture (thermoception), joint position (proprioception), body movement (kinaethesis), a full bladder, hunger or thirst, the ability to focus on a single voice in a room full of noise, and we even have a sense faculty that regulates the carbon-dioxide content in our blood. These senses contribute to the overall perception and understanding of the environment. This is why rewilding our senses through nature-based practices is so important.

Our senses should not be taken for granted. When we perceive our surroundings through our senses, we ground ourselves in the direct experience of life. Our bodily senses are a faculty that provides us with new knowledge about our circumstances and the environments we find ourselves in, but it also allows us to form a relationship with all the different dimensions of nature, and build new thoughts, ideas, and concepts.

Recognizing that our experiences are filtered through our bodies and senses has several implications for how we understand our personal experiences. Of particular importance is the recognition of the idea that our body is our 'instrument of communication' with the world, as nature extends an invitation to us to embrace her abundant offerings.

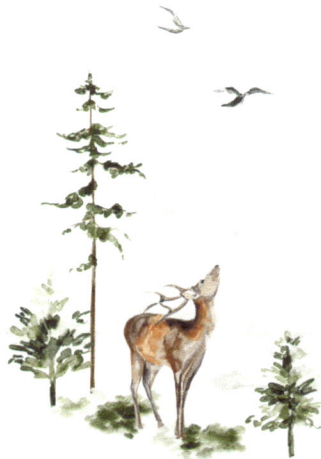

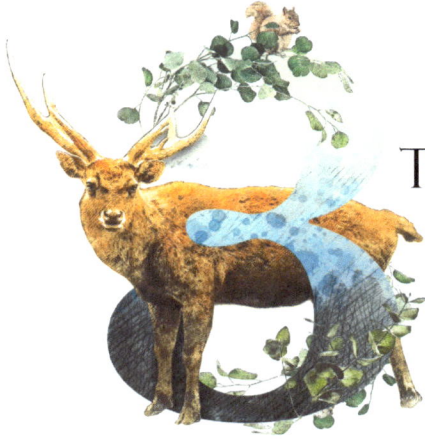

BEFORE WE BEGIN: THE DEFINITION OF 'SOUL'

The concept of the soul is multifaceted, encompassing a myriad of meanings that vary significantly among individuals and cultures. At its core, the soul is often perceived as the eternal, immaterial essence that defines a person's identity. It can embody consciousness, emotions, and individuality, transcending the boundaries of the physical body. In various belief systems and philosophies, the soul represents the seat of one's spirituality and connection to the divine or the sacred. It is a deeply personal and subjective aspect of human existence, inviting contemplation and exploration.

I will be using the term "soul" in the context of these nature therapy exercises to signify the following:

Soul is the innermost essence, an underlying ingredient, that allows for all things to have an internal dimension; no matter what shape it takes, no matter how simple or complex a system it is, it still has a hidden inner world. Through soul, all of life, including our living, breathing Earth, takes on a form, an essence, and enters our awareness—every sheltering tree, every resilient stone, every vitalizing drop of water. When we meet things on a soul level, the source of life itself, we illuminate our consciousness, boundaries wash away, and meaning is made possible. We give everyday experiences a fuller, richer, deeper significance.

Soul then moves from being a single possession for humans alone to being collective. Our awareness shifts from just being viewed as my soul, my fate, my biases to being interwoven within a living world, a larger soul, that encompasses our natural world. Nature now becomes an extension of ourselves. We awaken the rigidity of our minds to consider, to discover, that everything in our natural world is permeated with life, intelligence, and soul.

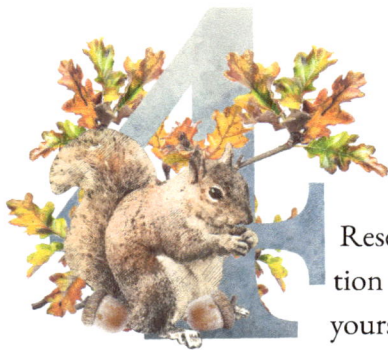

GETTING IN
THE RIGHT MINDSET

Research demonstrates that lasting and profound transformation is closely linked to experiences that are embodied.[14] Opening yourself up to experiencing all sensations, feelings, and thoughts within the body unlocks pathways to a holistic sense of wellbeing and to living a more meaningful life.

1. Take a moment to silence your phone. It's crucial that we maintain a quiet environment to allow everyone to fully engage with nature. Your cooperation in minimizing distractions will contribute to the overall success.

2. Be open and receptive. Be available to engaging and co-creating with your loving, intelligent heart energy and your imaginative capabilities.

3. The keys for our nature walk are intention and trust. State your intention, such as,

> "To rekindle my relationship with nature," "To find inner peace," or,
> "To experience healing within the natural world."

4. Breathe deeply. Slowly take your attention out of the external world, and move your attention within.

5. Allow yourself the space to contemplate the questions presented in each practice, letting your reflections and body's wisdom enrich your relationship with nature and your own internal landscape. These questions serve to anchor us in the present moment, acting as a bridge between our thoughts and our physical bodies. You're invited to embrace the insights as they come to light, so they may be fully lived, deeply breathed, and consciously carried forward in your life.

---

14   Bentz, J., do Carmo, L., Schafenacker, N. et al. "Creative, embodied practices, and the potentialities for sustainability transformations." Sustainability Science 17, 687–699 (2022). https://doi.org/10.1007/s11625-021-01000-2.

THE THRESHOLD

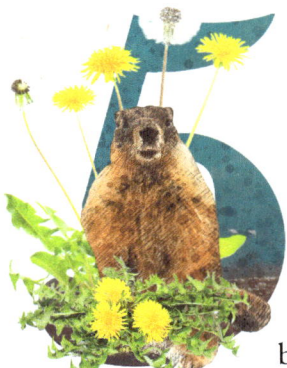

This moment is a threshold, a boundary symbolizing a deliberate transition from our world, the world that we know, into the world of the sacred or healing space. It's a place where humans and all beings come together without separations or differences. Crossing this threshold signifies a commitment to being fully present, open to the natural world, and receptive to the experience that follows. Each step along the path is a conscious choice to engage with nature.

In the context of nature-based therapy, thresholds can take various forms, each holding a unique significance. Here are a few different types of thresholds and their symbolic meanings:

1. Gateways: Physical entrances, such as the entrance to a forest or a garden, serve as literal gateways into nature. Crossing through a gateway can symbolize leaving behind the outside world and entering a sacred or healing space. It marks the beginning of a transformative experience.

2. Pathways: The start of a winding trail or a forest path can represent the beginning of a journey, both physically and metaphorically. Stepping onto a path signifies a commitment to exploring, learning, and being present.

3. Crossing Natural Features: Crossing over fallen logs, stepping stones in a stream, or small bridges can represent overcoming obstacles or challenges, or a transition from a busy or stressed mindset to a calmer, more mindful one.

4. Transitional Zones: Places where two different ecosystems meet, like the edge of a forest or the shore of a lake, can serve as powerful thresholds. These areas are rich in biodiversity and signify the harmony between different natural elements. Crossing these zones can symbolize embracing diversity and finding balance in one's own life.

6. Seasonal Changes: The changing of seasons, especially in deciduous forests, can create natural thresholds. Walking from an area of vibrant autumn foliage to a snowy winter landscape, for example, can represent the cyclical nature of life and the importance of adaptation and change.

In nature therapy, recognizing and acknowledging these different types of thresholds can enhance the therapeutic experience. They serve as reminders to be present, encouraging individuals to be mindful of their surroundings and the symbolic meanings attached to these natural markers.

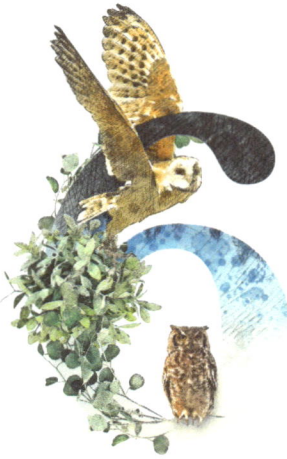

AT THE THRESHOLD:
A MINDFUL BREATH

Breathe in deeply, welcoming the gift of each moment; exhale, letting go of the past and stepping into the now. I invite you to close your eyes and engage all of your senses; to see, hear, touch, taste, smell, and feel.

Let the breeze delicately brush your skin, connecting you to the Earth beneath, syncing your heartbeat with nature's rhythm. Envision the sunlight filtering through the forest canopy, infusing your essence with its radiant glow. Allow its comforting warmth to thaw all your secret shields and defenses. There is no need for them in this sacred space.

Sense how the wind's airy touch envelops your presence, delicately sweeping through every cell in your body, taking with it all your thoughts, all your anxieties, all your concerns, and all your fears. To your surprise, they effortlessly slip away into the wind. In that moment, peace finds a home in your heart, and your mind embraces a soothing calm.

Take a moment to inhale deeply, savoring the freshness and innocence carried by the flora. Breathe in the peace and stillness provided by the trees.

Continue down the path.

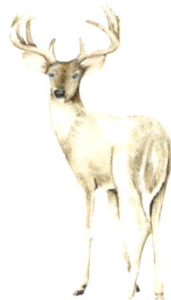

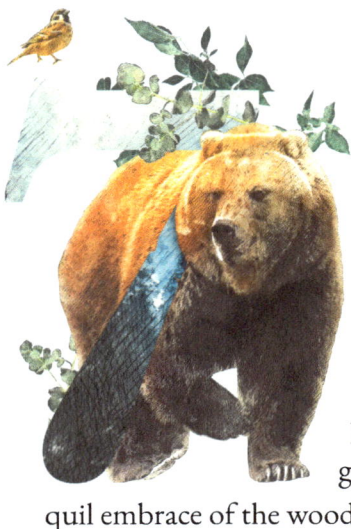

EMBRACING THE MOTION OF THE FOREST

Inhale deeply, syncing your breath with each purposeful step as you begin to walk slowly into the forest. Feel the subtle poetry of motion that surrounds you, intertwining with the rhythm of your breath. Exhale, letting go of the outside world, allowing the graceful movement of your steps to guide you deeper into the tranquil embrace of the woods.

Observe the leaves, like delicate ballerinas, gracefully swaying to the rhythm of the breeze, creating a mesmerizing spectacle of rustling melodies. Spider webs, masterpieces of intricacy, sway gently, capturing the sunlight in their gossamer threads. Pollinators, from bees to butterflies, engage in a lively choreography as they flit from flower to flower, contributing to the vibrant dance of nature. Flowers, in their myriad colors, bloom and nod in the gentle breeze, adding a splash of elegance to the landscape and enhancing the overall beauty of the harmonious scene. In this delicate ecosystem, dragonflies flit and dart, painting arcs of grace against the canvas of the forest. All the while birds, with masterful flights and melodic songs, paint the sky with their intricate patterns, completing the harmonious scene as they navigate through the serene landscape.

Amidst what may seem like stillness, you witness a vibrant world in constant motion. Each rustle, every gentle sway, and all fleeting movements weave together a tapestry pulsing with life. Allow the motion of the forest to stir your soul, inviting you to become one with the eternal rhythm of the natural world.

Allow yourself the space to contemplate the questions presented in each practice, letting your reflections enrich your relationship with the forest and your own emotional landscape.

As you witness this perpetual movement, how does it stir your emotions?

Does the motion of the forest evoke a sense of unity and relationships, or does it inspire awe at the meticulous choreography of existence?

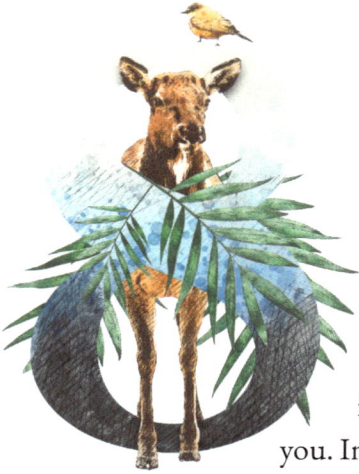

HARMONIZING WITH THE FOREST'S HEARTBEAT

Take a moment to stand still in the heart of the forest, acknowledging the gentle swaying of the trees, the fluttering leaves, and the subtle movements of the wildlife around you. Inhale deeply, absorbing the forest's unique scent, and exhale, releasing any tension. Allow your body to sway gently, syncing with the forest's rhythm.

1. Embrace the Rhythmic Dance

Observe the rhythmic dance of the forest—each tree, leaf, and creature moving in harmony with the wind's whispers. Each swaying branch and rustling plant tells a story of resilience and adaptation, a tale woven into the very fabric of the woodland symphony. Witness this mesmerizing choreography, an ageless dance that has played out through the centuries. As you observe, allow yourself to become attuned to the primal beat of nature, feeling the timeless energy that flows through the forest. Embrace this dance as a reminder of the interconnectedness of all living things, finding solace in the harmonious movements that echo the heartbeat of the Earth.

How did observing the forest's dance impact your own sense of rhythm and movement?

What emotions did you feel as you synchronized your movements with the swaying trees and falling leaves?

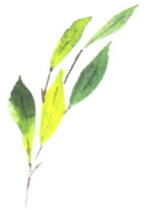

2. Engage Your Senses

Inhale mindfully, tuning into the ever-changing sensory elements that surround you. Exhale, freeing your mind from external distractions, allowing your senses to lead the way in this exploration.

Close your eyes and listen intently to the whispers of nature, connecting you with the natural pulse of the forest. Can you hear the rustle of leaves, the chirping of birds, or the patter of raindrops? Maybe the distant chatter of squirrels, the rhythmic tapping of a woodpecker, or the soft sigh of the wind through the trees reaches your ears. Imagine you can touch the movement around you, sensing the energy in the air. Extend your awareness to the gentle touch of leaves against your skin, the coolness of the breeze, or the textured bark of the trees, allowing the forest's tactile elements to further envelop your senses.

Open your eyes and witness the intricate details of the foliage, the velvety touch of moss-covered surfaces, and the kaleidoscope of colors exhibited by the diverse array of flowers. Take note of the subtle dance of sunlight on the forest floor, highlighting the beauty of each natural component. Allow your gaze to appreciate the nuanced textures, patterns, and hues, turning the forest into a gallery of captivating artistry waiting to be discovered. Now, deepen your experience. Inhale the earthy aroma, letting the forest's essence fill your lungs. Feel the subtle vibrations of the forest floor beneath your feet, grounding you in the ancient rhythm of nature. Allow the rich scents and tactile sensations to weave together, immersing yourself fully in the tapestry of the natural world around you, creating an unforgettable memory of nature's diverse wonders.

> Which sensory experience resonated with you the most—the rustle of leaves, the whispers of the wind, or the earthy aroma? Why?

> Reflect on how these sensations deepen your connection with the forest's motion.

3. Embracing Mutual Perception
Contemplate the remarkable understanding that the intelligent, living world is acutely aware, sensing our presence as keenly as, if not more so than, we sense it. Recognize that we are not passive observers but active participants, engaged in a reciprocal exchange with nature. We are perceived by the forest as deeply as we perceive it. As you absorb this awareness, feel the intricate threads of connection weaving you into the very soul of the forest, fostering a profound sense of belonging and mutual understanding.

> Contemplate the idea that the forest is aware of your presence. How does this awareness impact your understanding of your relationship with nature?

> Reflect on the concept of mutual experience. In what ways do you believe the forest experiences your presence and emotions?

> How can the understanding of mutual perception between humans and nature influence your future interactions with the natural world?

4. Connect with Flowing Water
If there's a creek, stream, or brook nearby, approach its flowing waters. Observe how the water moves effortlessly, creating intricate patterns and ripples. Listen to its soothing melody and feel its cool embrace. Acknowledge the water's constant motion as a

reminder of life's continuous flow.

> How did witnessing the water's flow affect your understanding of
> emotional fluidity and adaptability?

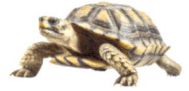

> Consider the emotions that surfaced as you observed the water's journey.
> How do these emotions relate to your own experiences of change and transition?

5. Animal Encounters

Pay attention to the forest's inhabitants in motion. Whether it's a squirrel darting up a tree, a bird taking flight, or an ant crossing your path, observe their agility and grace. Reflect on how these creatures navigate their surroundings with such finesse, finding purpose in every movement. Marvel at their adaptability and learn from their seamless connection with nature.

> Which forest creature's motion resonated with you the most, and why?

> How can you embody the grace and purpose of these forest creatures
> in your own movements and actions?

> Reflect on the emotions you sensed in the animals' movements.
> How did their behaviors mirror or contrast your own emotional states?

6. Silent Observations

Witness the play of light filtering through the forest canopy, casting ever-shifting patterns on the ground. Observe how the dancing sunlight creates a symphony of shadows and illuminates the path before you. Notice the emotional response within you as the forest's mood shifts with the changing light. Embrace the dynamic interplay between light and shadow, acknowledging the emotional resonance it evokes.

> How did the shifting light patterns influence your emotional state?
> Did certain patterns evoke specific feelings?

> How does the fleeting nature of light and shadow encourage you to
> appreciate the present moment more fully?

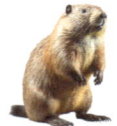

> Are there aspects of yourself that you tend to conceal in the shadows, and how
> might acknowledging them bring more balance and acceptance into your life?

7. Emotional Resonance

In the quietude of the forest, acknowledge the resonance of your emotions. Feel the joy of a bird's song, the peace of a gently swaying branch, and the excitement of a rustling squirrel. Recognize how your own emotions echo in response. Embrace this resonance, understanding that your feelings are not isolated but connected to the intricate web of life around you.

How did the forest's emotional resonance reflect or amplify your own emotions?

Consider the variety of emotions you experienced. Did any particular emotion surprise you, and why?

8. Aromatic Serenity

Take a slow, deliberate breath in, savoring the forest air, and attune your senses to the subtle aromas gently transported by the wind. With each exhale, let go of stress, allowing the natural fragrances to become a soothing part of your inhalation and exhalation.

Breath in slowly, capturing the scent of the ancient trees, the moss-covered rocks, the subtle flowers in bloom, the lacy fronds of ferns, the earthy woodland floor, and the crisp, invigorating air that defines the unique aroma of the forest. Allow the rich tapestry of scents in the forest to unfold with each inhalation.

Notice how these scents transform and mingle with the changing winds, creating a fragrant journey through the forest. Reflect on the specific scents that resonate with your senses and consider how they may contribute to the rejuvenation and healing of your body.

As you breathe in the healing aromas, visualize the energy of the forest merging with your own. How does this visualization enhance your overall sense of well-being and connection with nature?

As you inhale these forest aromas, how does your breathing pattern change?

Consider the harmony of different aromas blending together in the forest. How does this blend of scents influence your sensory experience and emotional response?

Reflect on the transformative power of aroma in motion. In what ways do these scents help you release stress and embrace a sense of peace, both physically and mentally?

9. Eternal Resonance

Wander through the natural surroundings until a particular stone catches your eye, one that resonates with you. Feel the energy of the stone beneath your fingertips. As you absorb the essence of the stone, imagine yourself becoming one with it, grounding your energy and consciousness in its timeless existence. Spend a few moments in this stone-like stillness, observing the world from this unyielding perspective. Hold close to your heart the profound understanding that, like the enduring stone, the essence you leave behind in this life has the potential to echo through eternity. Allow this realization to inspire a sense of heart-centered connection to the enduring rhythms of the natural world and a deep recognition of the lasting impact of your own energy and presence.

> How does the tactile experience of feeling the energy of the stone beneath your fingertips contribute to a heightened sense of embodiment and connection with the natural world?

> As you hold the understanding that the essence you leave behind has the potential to echo through eternity, how does this realization manifest in your physical being? Consider any sensations or movements within your body that reflect this profound understanding.

10. Soul of the Forest

Inhale the sacred breath of the forest, inviting the spirit of nature to intertwine with your own, and as you exhale, release any tensions, forging a profound connection with the soulful energy that resides within the heart of the woods.

As you delve deeper into the forest's heart, sense the soul of the woods—the timeless soul that breathes life into every leaf, creature, and stone. Feel its ancient wisdom, a reservoir of knowledge and serenity. In this profound connection, recognize the interwoven tapestry of souls—the trees, the animals, and your own. Acknowledge the eternal bond that unites all living beings. Reflect on how this connection enriches your understanding of the world and deepens your appreciation for the intricate dance of life.

> What emotions arise when you imagine the ancient soul of the forest? How does this awareness affect your own sense of time and existence?

> Consider the wisdom you feel emanating from the forest's soul. In what ways can you integrate this wisdom into your own life?

Reflect on the tranquility of the forest's soul. How does this calmness compare to your usual state of mind?

Closing

Hold within you the emotional depth and soulful bond you've shared with the forest. Extend your heartfelt appreciation to the forest and all its moving wonders. Honor the soulful dance of leaves, the gentle whispers of the wind, and the fragrant symphony that caresses your senses. Gratitude fills your heart for the healing aromas that touch your soul, leading you toward profound inner peace and wellbeing. With reverence, you acknowledge the intricate choreography of the forest in motion, a testament to the soulful essence of nature. May this deep gratitude stay with you, nurturing your connection to the forest and inspiring you to protect its beauty for generations to come.

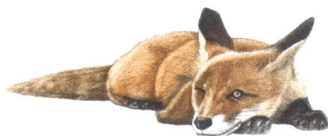

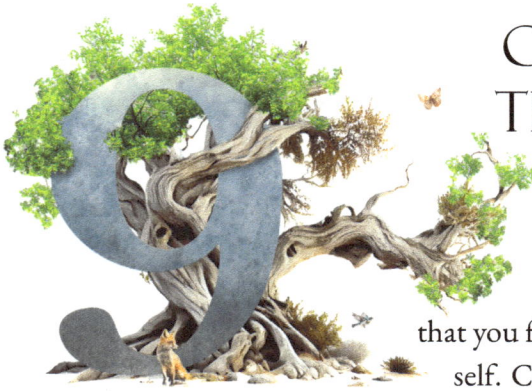

COMMUNING WITH THE ANCIENT TREE: DEEP FEELING

Find a quiet corner within the forest, near a tree that you feel drawn to, and take a moment to ground yourself. Close your eyes gently, allowing the natural sounds of the forest to envelop you. Breathe deeply, inhaling the earthy aroma that surrounds you, connecting with the very essence of the forest. Now, slowly open your eyes and direct your attention to the magnificent, ancient tree before you. This tree, a sentinel of time, stands tall and wise, its roots firmly embedded in the earth, its branches reaching out to touch the sky.

1. Engage Your Senses

Direct your focus toward the age-old tree standing in front of you. Gaze upon its gnarled bark, silently seeking permission to touch it. Move closer, allowing your hands to explore its surface. Feel the rugged texture beneath your fingertips, tracing the cracks and crevices, gently touching the leaves, and running your hands along its branches.

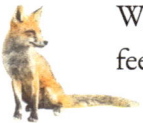

> What visual characteristics and textures do you observe? How do these textures feel to the touch?

> Are there any specific patterns or roughness that stand out? Compare this texture with other trees nearby. In what ways does it differ?

> How might these differences serve a purpose in the tree's natural environment?

2. Sense Its Presence

As your hands move across the bark, pay attention to the sensations rippling through your fingers, arms, and body.

> How does touching the tree make its presence known throughout your being?

3. Connect with its Role in Nature

Imagine the tree as a haven for birds, butterflies, bats, moths, ants, and squirrels. Envision it as a sanctuary for countless beings that have traveled long distances and seek refuge under its branches. Consider the tree's vital role in the intricate web of life supporting these Earthborn companions as they do their work in the world.

What emotions arise within you as you contemplate its significance in the ecosystem?

4. Feel the Earth Beneath Your Feet

Take off your shoes and connect with the earth beneath the tree. Curl your toes into the soil. Is it hard, soft, moist, or dry? Visualize the tree's essence flowing from its roots, up its trunk, and into its branches. Feel the subtle warmth or coolness of its energy.

How does this connection change your experience with the tree? Notice what your heart is telling you.

5. Inhale the Tree's Gift

Inhale deeply, imagining the tree offering you its life-giving oxygen and healing compounds. Picture the oxygen flowing from the leaves above, traveling down into your lungs, and circulating through your body.

How does the oxygen feel as it enters your lungs? What sensations accompany each breath? Can you discern any unique flavors or scents in the air?

Now, take a deep breath in through your mouth. What sensations accompany the air entering your lungs? Are there any variations in the scent that you can identify?

6. Acknowledge the Sacred Exchange

Reflect on the sacred exchange occurring between you and the tree. As you breathe out, visualize your words of gratitude and reverence carried on the molecules of your breath, reaching the tree and becoming a part of its essence.

How does it feel to know you're sharing this intimate connection with the tree?

7. Listen and Receive
Take a moment to listen to the ancient tree.

> What wisdom does it share?

> What thoughts, emotions, or memories arise within you as you connect with its ancient energy?

8. Reflect on Centuries of Wisdom
Imagine the hundreds of years this tree has stood in that place. Contemplate the experiences, stories, and lives it has witnessed: children climbing its branches, travelers resting beneath its shade, wars and migrations unfolding around it, and the changing landscape. Consider its wisdom, patience, and enduring capacity.

> What emotions are stirred within you as you acknowledge the tree's profound journey through time?

9. Embodying Existence
Beneath the forest's verdant canopy, where sunlight filters through a mosaic of foliage, casting shifting patterns on the forest floor, let's honor the principle that we don't speak of trees aging, but rather of their eternal growth. Deepen and slow your breath, inviting it to venture deeply into the sanctuary of your heart. Breathe in the essence of life itself, the earthy scent rising from the soil enveloping you.

As you exhale, extend this same reverence to yourself, recognizing that you are not simply aging, but blossoming into the fullness of your being. Like the tree, celebrate your continuous growth, each leaf unfurling, each root delving deeper, in an ever-unfolding journey of growth, vitality, and discovery.

> How can you cultivate a mindset that celebrates your continuous growth, much like the unfurling leaves and deepening roots of the trees in the forest?

> In what ways can you embrace the essence of life within yourself, mirroring the earthy scent rising from the soil?

Reflecting on the shifting patterns of sunlight within the forest, how can you adapt to life's ever-changing circumstances with grace and resilience?

10. Soulful Connection with Nature

Acknowledge the soulful connection between your essence and the heartbeat of the forest. Envision your soul intertwining with the ancient souls of this tree and the very earth beneath your feet. Consider the wisdom ingrained in the tree's silence and the messages whispered by the rustling leaves. Reflect on the shared essence of life, recognizing that your existence is harmoniously woven into the fabric of nature.

Contemplate the profound sense of belonging that permeates your being as you listen deeply, transcending the boundaries between your soul and the soul of the tree.

Closing

Offer your heartfelt thanks to the tree for its presence, its oxygen, and its wisdom. Imagine your words being absorbed by the tree, becoming a part of its story. Know that you have shared a sacred moment with a living being that has witnessed centuries of life. Carry this connection with you, letting it nourish your soul and inspire your journey. As you step away, express your gratitude once more and continue your path, carrying the ancient tree's wisdom within your heart.

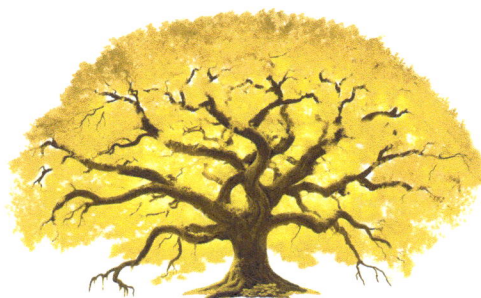

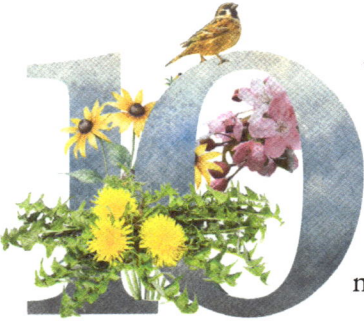

THE FOREST SOUNDSCAPE: DEEP LISTENING

Nature is rich with a symphony of sounds. However, our busy minds frequently overlook the sights and sounds that envelop us.

Sound is part of our memory. It has a physicality that allows us to be utterly present or transported to a special place. The manner in which we listen plays a pivotal role in shaping the quality of our interactions and contributes significantly to generating new experiences.

Deep listening allows us to see through the eyes of another, and connect with their experience. Apart from listening for facts, we listen for what is different. We listen with our minds and hearts wide open, receptive to an interaction between our senses and the surrounding environment. Deep listening is a heart-to-heart interaction. We shift our awareness to letting go of what we know and surrender to just listening for no other purpose than to hear an-other. We listen for more than is consciously spoken. We listen in order to give an-other a voice, a chance to be heard, and thereby, maybe, suffer less. Please keep in mind, even silence can appear to others like all is right.

Find a comfortable spot to sit or stand in the heart of the forest. Begin by gently closing your eyes or softening your gaze. Release any tension in your body and allow your arms to rest naturally by your sides, letting go of any belongings you might be carrying.

Take a deep breath, embracing the delightful, crisp fragrances of this remarkable place. Breathe in fully, embracing the energy of life; exhale, allowing yourself to merge seamlessly with its unfolding journey.

1. Embrace the Soundscape

Tune in to the natural symphony surrounding you. Let your awareness open to the chorus of animals, insects, and birds. Feel the caress of the wind against your skin. What sounds do you discern?

> Are there creatures moving in the underbrush, leaves rustling in the breeze, or distant calls of birds?

2. Engage Your Senses

Shift your attention to the physicality of sound. Notice how it has a tangible presence, connecting you deeply to the present moment. Feel the vibrations of the forest sounds resonating within you.

What emotions do these vibrations evoke?

3. Deep Listening with Animals

Animals, the masters of deep listening, are fully present in their surroundings; honor their attentive nature. Consider how they might perceive and understand the forest soundscape differently than you. Imagine the wisdom in their stillness, and how they embrace the forest symphony long before you notice their presence. Reflect on the interconnectedness between their attentive ears and the natural world.

How does this awareness shift your perception of their silent presence?

4. Explore the Layers of Sound

Focus on the sounds surrounding you. Can you distinguish different layers of sounds? Pay attention to subtle or distant noises that might have escaped your notice before. Notice how the combination of these sounds create a unique atmosphere.

How do these auditory cues shape your overall experience? Do they evoke specific emotions or deepen your connection with the forest?

5. Change in Perspective

Rotate 90 degrees to either your left or right. Observe how the soundscape transforms. Notice the nuances in the sounds, the altered rhythm of the forest symphony.

How does your experience shift now that you've changed direction? How does this change in perspective enhance your connection with the environment?

6. Heighten Your Hearing

Enhance the forest sounds by softly cupping your hands behind your ears. Stay attentive to the delicate forest noises enveloping you. Direct your focus towards sounds that capture your interest. Explore the depth of each tone and its resonance within the forest. Reflect on the significance of these captured sounds in amplifying your sensory experience.

Why do these sounds capture your attention?

What are you feeling within your body as you listen?

7. Connect with a Specific Animal

Take a deep, slow breath, allowing the forest air to fill your lungs. Once again, attune your senses to the symphony of sounds surrounding you. Engage your curiosity and focus on a specific animal in your vicinity. Observe its behavior.

Does he appear to notice you? Is he singing or chattering with a friend, feeling threatened, or just enjoying the day? Pay attention to the nuances in the tone and pitch of his sounds.

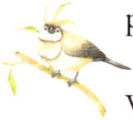

With intent and deep understanding, immerse yourself in the animal's vocalizations or movements. It could be his voice, the movement of his wings, or the sound of his movement, like the tapping of a woodpecker. Try to vocalize the sound using your own syllables, encouraging a profound level of attentive listening. For example: a frog may say, ga-ruck, ga-ruck, or you hear the zizza-zeez from the wings of a dragon fly. This exercise challenges you to listen with heightened awareness and connect deeply with the forest's inhabitants.

8. Heightened Awareness

With your heightened hearing, explore unfamiliar sounds in the forest. Is the sound in motion? If so, can you determine its origin and destination? Engage with the mystery of these unfamiliar sounds, following their trajectories through the forest. Notice the interplay between these sounds and the natural environment, and how your heightened awareness enriches your connection with the unseen life within the forest.

For a moment, engage with the farthest sound audible to your ears.

Now, redirect your focus to the nearest sound in your immediate surroundings.

What is it like to merge with the soundscape enveloping you?

9. Explore the Silence

Amidst the sounds, notice the moments of silence. Silence can be as expressive as sound, holding the unspoken language of the forest. Embrace the tranquility and breathe in the serenity of the quiet intervals.

What does the silence reveal to you about the forest's essence?

What sensations arise when immersed in silence?

How does your body respond to this quietude?

10. Merge with the Soundscape

Merge your breath with the soundscape. Inhale deeply, allowing the forest air to fill your lungs. Notice how your breath synchronizes with the rhythms of the forest. Feel your heartbeat aligning with the natural cadence of the surroundings.

How does this harmonious connection affect your sense of presence?

11. Focus on Heart-Centered Listening

Shift your attention to your heart center. Imagine your heartbeats echoing the forest's pulse. Listen not only with your ears but also with your heart. Feel the resonance between your heart's energy and the energy of the forest.

What emotions arise within you as your heart connects with nature's heartbeat?

Closing

Carry this profound experience of deep listening with you. The forest has shared its symphony, its intricate language, its secrets, and its silence. Let this awareness stay with you, reminding you of the interconnectedness between all living beings. Let your gratitude reverberate through the forest, a silent acknowledgment of the sacred exchange between you and the natural world.

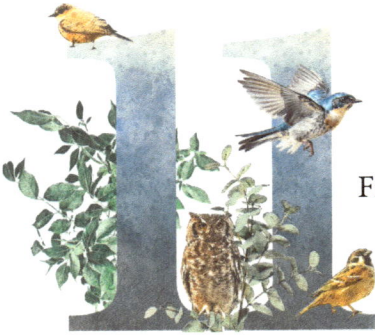

SYMPHONY IN FEATHERS: DEEP LISTENING

Find a quiet spot in the heart of the forest. Sit or stand comfortably, grounding yourself in the natural surroundings. Close your eyes gently and take a few deep breaths, allowing yourself to tune in to the soundscape around you. In this moment, your focus will be on listening deeply to the diverse melodies of the birds that make their home in this forest.

1. Focus on One Birdsong

Start by concentrating on the song of a single bird. Let its melody draw you in, and become attuned to its rhythm, pitch, and tone. Listen to its song as if it were a message from nature, communicating with just you.

What emotions or sensations arise as you listen to the birds in the forest?

2. Expand Your Awareness

Gradually expand your awareness to include other bird calls around you. Notice how each bird has its unique voice, contributing to the symphony of the forest. Observe the harmonious interplay between the different sounds.

How do the various birdsongs make you feel?

As you notice the different bird calls around you, how do these diverse sounds contribute to the overall ambiance of the forest?

Are there particular bird melodies that resonate more profoundly with your emotions or memories?

3. Embrace the Silence

In between the birdsongs, embrace the moments of silence. Let the quietude deepen your listening experience. Silence, too, is a significant part of the forest's melody.

How does the experience of deep listening to birdsongs enhance your connection with nature and your sense of presence in the forest?

4. Feel the Vibrations

Pay attention not just to the auditory sensations but also to the vibrations. Feel the subtle vibrations of the birdsongs resonating within you, connecting you to the pulse of nature.

> Reflecting on the subtle vibrations of the birdsongs, did you find a harmony between the vibrations and your own inner state?

5. Soulful Connection with Birdsongs

Do you notice a soulful connection, more than just the auditory experience? You may feel a sense of harmony, peace, or even a spiritual alignment with the birdsongs. It's as if the songs speak to something deep within you, touching your innermost emotions, thoughts, or spiritual beliefs.

> In what ways did the birdsongs resonate with your soul or inner being? Did you sense a deeper connection beyond the auditory experience, perhaps on a spiritual or emotional level?

> How might this connection influence your understanding of your place in the natural world?

Breathe. Hear the birds' tender songs as they invite your soul to take flight in the vast expanse of their soul-nourishing choir. Visualize your soul radiating with light, then allow it to ascend upwards and soar on the notes of their sweet, unforgettable melodies. Give your soul time to sing along with the birds, ride the wind's currents, to explore, to play, to enjoy.

Closing

Take a moment to offer your thanks for the gifts of this experience. Allow the melodies of the forest to weave themselves into the fabric of your being. Let the songs of the birds echo in your heart, a reminder of the intricate harmony of nature. With each chirp and trill, you have touched a chord within yourself, resonating with the essence of nature. As you step back into the world beyond the trees, may the echoes of these bird songs guide you, a constant reminder of the beauty and interconnectedness of all life.

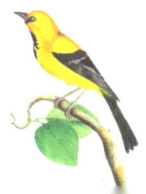

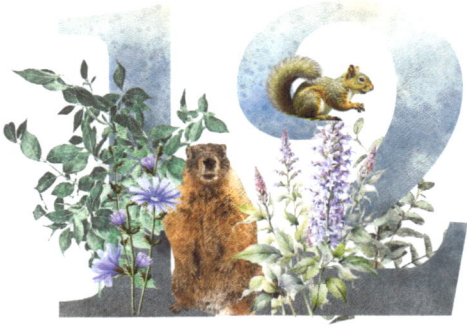

A PLAYFUL SPIRIT: DEEP ATTENTION

Within this nature experience, we embrace the power of deep attention and playful imagination to connect with nature.

What do you normally notice in nature when you are out for a walk? If you take a few minutes to watch how your mind works and what you've been perceiving, you'll likely notice how unconscious your observations are. Typically, we don't consciously choose what we observe. Most of us tend to concentrate on what lies directly ahead, or where we're walking, only diverting our gaze when something grabs our interest. Yet, when you pause to glance around, you frequently discover things that previously escaped your attention or didn't register in your awareness.

For a few moments, inhale deeply, embracing the pure and invigorating scents of this enchanting place. Breathe in life to its fullest; exhale, surrendering to the moment.

1. Embracing the Marvels of Nature

Take a moment to open your awareness wide, like the petals of a blooming flower in the morning sun. Imagine your senses awakening, tuning in to the subtle symphony of nature that surrounds you.

Now, softly close your eyes, shutting out the external world, and let your consciousness delve into the realm of your inner senses. Feel the gentle caress of the breeze on your skin, sense the earthy aroma rising from the ground beneath you, and hear the soft whispers of leaves rustling in the wind. In this stillness, visualize the world around you, painted in the vibrant hues of the natural landscape.

After a few moments, open your eyes, allowing the outside world to seep in. Notice the dance of sunlight filtering through the canopy, casting intricate patterns on the forest floor. Observe the intricate web of life, from the delicate veins on a leaf to the complex ecosystems thriving around you. As you breathe, let the fragrant whispers of blooming flowers and the musky scents of the earth fill your lungs.

Nature is not merely a backdrop but an intricate tapestry of life, eager to form a profound connection with you. Let your senses mingle with the environment, becoming attuned to the symphony of nature's sounds, textures, and fragrances, embracing this profound connection. As you open your awareness, you invite the wonders of nature to weave their magic, enveloping you in their timeless embrace.

Reflect on any emotions or thoughts that arose during this practice.

How do you think these feelings relate to your relationship with nature?

2. Embracing Playfulness

Recall the playful imagination of childhood. As adults, we don't often allow ourselves to be playful, imaginative, lighthearted, or just a little bit silly.

Now, in pairs, assume roles: one as the 'parent observer' and the other as the 'blind child'. Engage your imagination, be lighthearted, and describe the scene vividly.

Parents, please paint a detailed picture for the blind child, enabling them to visualize and experience nature through your words. Remember that nature's beauty is not confined solely to what we see. Engage the blind child's senses. Direct them to touch the ground, smell the flowers, feel the softness of the grass, and listen to the howl of coyotes or the whisper of the wind. Blind children, immerse yourselves in this vision, using your inner senses to perceive every detail. Experience the sounds, scents, and textures of the natural world.

Now repeat the activity, but this time switch roles: the parent observer takes on the role of the blind child, and vice versa.

3. Reflecting on the Experience

After the exercise, find a moment of stillness. Take deep breaths and acknowledge what you experienced anew. Reflect on the emotions that surfaced.

Did any specific memories or sensations arise?

Where in your body did you feel these emotions?

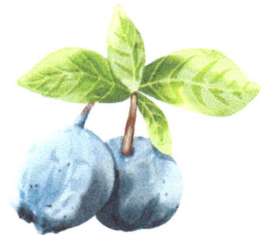

Closing

In the quietude of nature's embrace, express gratitude for the gifts of deep attention and playfulness that have woven a bit of nature's wonder into our senses. As you step away from this sacred moment, let the echoes of birdsong and the rustle of leaves remind you of the profound connections you've forged—with the natural world and within yourself. Carry the spirit of curiosity and attentiveness into your days, letting the playful dance of nature guide your senses and enrich your existence. Cherish the memories of this immersive, playful experience, allowing it to infuse your life with enduring wonder and awe.

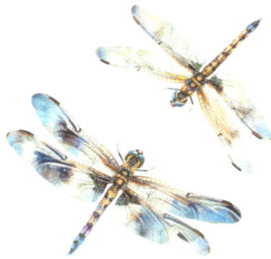

EXPLORING THE TEXTURES OF THE FOREST

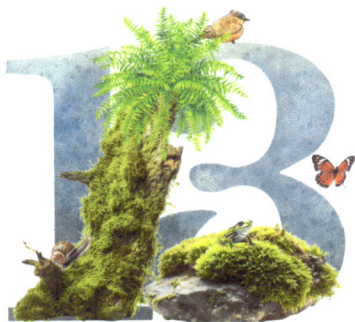

Find a serene spot in the heart of the forest. Sit or stand comfortably, grounding yourself in the natural surroundings. Close your eyes gently and take a few deep breaths. Inhale the earthy aroma of the forest, letting your senses attune to the sounds, scents, and textures around you. Open your eyes and let your gaze wander.

1. Touch the Rough Bark of a Tree

Approach a nearby tree and run your fingers over its rough bark. Feel the ancient texture beneath your fingertips. Notice the grooves, knots, and patterns. Sense the resilience of the tree and how it has weathered the passage of time.

> As your fingers trace the grooves, knots, and patterns on the tree's bark, consider how the scars and rugged textures tell the story of the tree's journey. How does this tactile experience remind you of life's challenges and the strength required to overcome obstacles?

> How can you draw inspiration from the tree's resilience for your own life?

2. Explore the Softness of Moss

Look for patches of moss beneath the trees. Gently touch the moss with your hand, feeling its softness and delicate structure. Observe how it provides a plush cushion, a testament to nature's intricate design.

> Experience the contrast between the rough bark and the velvety moss.

3. Feel the Smoothness of Leaves

Reach out and touch the leaves of different plants. Experience the smoothness of some leaves and the serrated edges of others. Pay attention to the variations in texture and thickness. Notice how each leaf has its unique surface, adapted for its purpose in the forest.

How can the appreciation of these textures inspire a deeper sense of respect and gratitude for the intricate tapestry of life in the forest?

4. Encounter the Coarseness of Stones

Find a stone or pebble on the forest floor. Run your fingers over its surface, feeling the coarseness and solidity. Contemplate the strength and endurance represented by the stone. Sense the ancient energy it holds, connecting you to the geological history of the forest and the Earth.

Notice the textures of rocks and stones, shaped by ancient forces and weathered by time. How do these sturdy textures evoke a sense of stability and endurance, grounding you in the present moment?

5. Dip Your Fingers in a Stream

If there's a nearby stream, dip your fingers into the flowing water. Feel the cool, refreshing sensation as the water flows around your skin. Experience the smoothness of the wet rocks beneath the surface.

Reflect on the fluidity and adaptability represented by the water.

6. Explore the Fuzziness of Lichens

Look for lichens growing on tree branches or rocks. Gently touch the fuzzy, velvety texture of lichens. Observe their unique patterns and colors. Contemplate the symbiotic relationship between fungi and algae, marveling at nature's ability to create harmony in diverse textures.

Reflect on the unique patterns and colors of the lichens you observe. How does this visual experience inspire a sense of awe and wonder about the creativity of nature?

7. Feel the Delicacy of Petals

If there are blooming flowers, delicately touch the petals. Experience the softness and fragility of the petals beneath your fingertips. Notice the vibrant colors and intricate patterns. Reflect on the transient beauty of flowers and the significance of appreciating the fleeting moments in life.

Reflect on the contrast between textures, such as the sharpness of thorns against the smoothness of petals. How does this interplay of rough and soft textures symbolize the balance and diversity within nature?

8. Experience the Richness of the Soil

Kneel down and gently touch the earth beneath the forest canopy. Feel the moist, fertile soil teeming with life. Let the soil sift through your fingers, connecting you to the ancient cycles of growth and decay. Reflect on the nourishing essence of the soil, sustaining the entire forest ecosystem.

> Consider the overall experience of immersing yourself in the textures, sounds, and scents of the forest. How has this nature exercise influenced your perspective on nature and its interconnectedness?

> How can you carry the wisdom of these sensory experiences into your daily life?

9. Sense the Gentle Caress of the Wind

Feel the wind as it brushes against your skin. Notice its varying intensity, from a gentle caress to a playful breeze. Observe how it carries whispers of the forest, connecting you with the unseen life around you. Allow the wind to remind you of the constant movement and energy in nature.

> How do these tactile sensations awaken your sense of touch and connection to nature?

10. Observe the Playful Dance of Clouds

Look up at the sky and observe the clouds drifting by. Notice their shapes, sizes, and the way they filter sunlight. Contemplate the vastness of the sky and the sense of freedom that comes with watching the ever-changing patterns of the clouds. Let your imagination wander with them.

11. Feel the Warmth of Sunlight Through Trees

Stand or sit in a patch of sunlight filtering through the trees. Close your eyes and feel the warmth on your skin. Notice the interplay of light and shadow, creating a dappled pattern on the forest floor. Allow the sunlight to evoke a sense of comfort and vitality within you.

12. Inhale the Aromas of the Forest

Take deep breaths and inhale the rich, earthy scents of the forest. Notice the subtle fragrances of pine, damp soil, and blooming flowers. Let the natural aromas fill your lungs and invigorate your senses. Connect with the forest through its distinct and rejuvenating smells.

Reflect on the interplay between the textures, sounds, and scents of the forest. How do these sensory experiences complement and enhance one another?

How can you incorporate a multi-sensory approach to enhance your mindfulness and presence in everyday life?

13. Listen to the Symphony of Forest Life

Tune in to the sounds of birds chirping, squirrels rustling in the trees, and crawling bugs and insects going about their daily activities. Allow the natural symphony to envelop you, filling your ears with the melodies of the forest. Observe how each sound contributes to the harmonious rhythm of the ecosystem.

Reflect on the sounds of birds and squirrels. How might their songs and chatter inspire you to embrace joy, playfulness, and communication in your own interactions?

14. Connect with the Soul of the Forest

Close your eyes and imagine the very soul of the forest. Feel its ancient wisdom, its quiet strength, and its nurturing presence. Sense the interconnectedness of all living beings within this sacred space. Acknowledge the soulful energy that envelops you, holding you in its eternal embrace.

Closing

Express gratitude for the forest and its teachings. Acknowledge the interconnectedness you share with all living beings and the Earth. Carry the peace of the forest with you as you continue your day, and may the sensory memories of this experience guide you back to nature whenever you need solace, inspiration, or a reminder of the beauty that surrounds us.

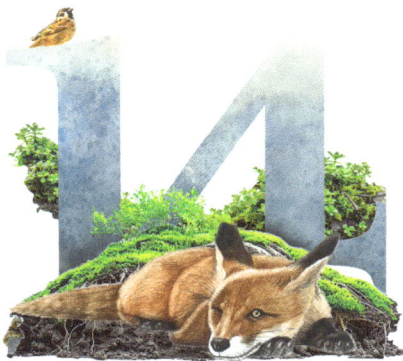

EARTHLY COMMUNION: A SOIL-CENTERED PRACTICE

Embarking on a profound journey of immersing your hands into the earth is more than a mere tactile exploration; it is a sacred communion with the very essence of life. In this nature-based practice, each intentional touch becomes a conduit for a deeper connection, an opportunity to intertwine your existence with the ancient soul of the world embedded in the soil. As you enter this sacred space, the act of placing your hands into the earth transcends the physical; it becomes a contemplative relationship between self and nature, an act of reverence for the sustaining forces that bind us to the intricate tapestry of the natural world.

Find a tranquil outdoor sanctuary that resonates with your spirit. Meander through the embrace of nature, seeking a space where the symphony of the elements harmonizes and beckons you into a state of serene connection. As you navigate through this exploration, attune yourself to the subtle shifts in the environment—the interplay of sunlight filtering through leaves, the gentle whispers of the wind, and the diverse palette of colors that grace the surroundings. Choose a space where the tranquility is palpable, providing a canvas for introspection and communion with the natural world. Once you arrive, find a patch of soil within this sacred space, whether it's a secluded garden, a peaceful woodland nook, or any corner where the Earth welcomes your presence.

1. Breath and Presence

Choose to sit, squat, or kneel in a position close to the ground that feels comfortable for you. Take in the visual details of the soil, envisioning the inhalation of the planet's essence with each breath. Inhale, drawing in the energy that courses through the soil, connecting you with the heartbeat of Earth herself. Exhale, letting go of any lingering stress or discord, and offer these remnants back to the nurturing soil of the Earth, where they may transform into beauty. This reciprocal exchange of breath aligns your essence with the Earth's vitality, fostering a profound unity in the shared rhythm of inhalation and exhalation.

2. Connection with Earth

Begin by gently touching the soil with your fingertips. If the soil is covered, gently move aside any leaves or debris to expose the bare earth. Run your fingers through the earth, allowing yourself to fully experience the sensations. Feel its temperature, moisture, and texture. Let your hands explore the variations in the earth, noting any stones, roots, or other natural elements. Further immerse your hands deeper into the earth and visualize a connection forming between yourself and the planet. Envision the energy of the Earth flowing through your fingertips, fostering a sense of unity and oneness with the natural world.

3. Mindful Movements

Move your hands intentionally through the soil, embracing a rhythmic and mindful pace. Consider the cyclical nature of life as you touch upon the cycles of growth, decay, and renewal.

4. Engage your senses

Open yourself completely to the full spectrum of sensory delights present in your surroundings. Observe the rich palette of colors and captivating patterns present in the soil. Listen with intent to the gentle rustling of leaves and the harmonious chorus of birdsong. Inhale slowly and deliberately, savoring the distinctive fragrance of the earth. Let these sensory impressions weave together, nurturing a connection within you that transcends the superficial, reaching into the depths of both your soul and the essence of the natural world.

> As you immerse your hands into the soil, how does the physical contact with the earth translate into sensations within your body? Are there specific points of connection or resonance that you can feel in your hands, arms, or even beyond?

5. Reflective journey into the soul of the soil

In the act of touching the soil, allow your thoughts to unfold and dwell on the sustenance it graciously bestows upon every living entity—humans, plants, animals, and the entire ecosystem. Reflect on the profound interconnectedness of life, recognizing the vital role played by the soil in sustaining the intricate balance of nature, and appreciate your role as a steward within this interwoven fabric of existence.

6. Expressive Connection

Should you be moved to do so, express your thoughts or feelings verbally. Share words of appreciation, gratitude, or perhaps poetry, creating an opportunity to further deepen your connection with the Earth and the vitalizing energy it generously provides.

7. Carry the Earth with You

Before leaving, gently gather a small amount of soil in your hands, allowing the earth to rest in your palms. Carry this precious handful of soil with you, placing it in a pocket or a small container. Let it become a reminder of the profound connection forged during this practice. When you need grounding throughout the day, revisit the sensation of the earth in your hands. View it as a source of strength, a symbol of the enduring bond between yourself and the natural world. In this simple yet profound act, you carry with you the grounding essence of the Earth, providing a touchstone for tranquility and a reconnection to the profound beauty that exists in the simplicity of nature.

> As you engage in the soil practice, how does the awareness of the interconnected relationship between humans, plants, animals, and the soil itself influence your understanding of your role in sustaining the delicate balance of life on Earth?

Closing

As you prepare to conclude this nature-inspired experience, extend your heartfelt gratitude to the Earth for the boundless energy and unwavering support she generously shares with you. Whether you choose to stand or sit, take a deliberate moment to bask in this sense of appreciation. Feel the resonance of your thanks reverberate through the connection you've cultivated, acknowledging the harmonious exchange between yourself and the nurturing forces of the Earth.

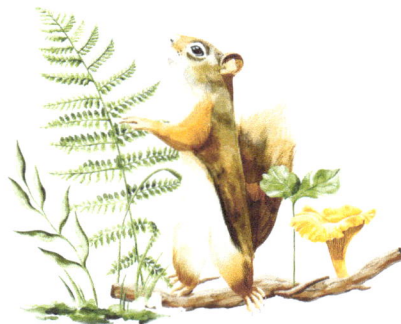

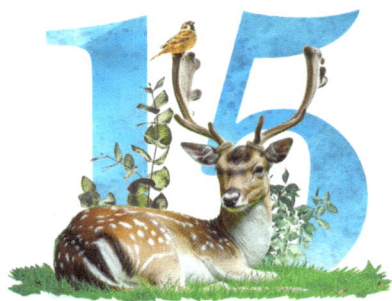

FINDING PEACE IN WATER'S PRESENCE

Before immersing yourself in the tranquil embrace of water, take a moment to prepare your senses and connect with the natural rhythm of your breath. Inhale deeply, allowing the forest air to fill your lungs, infusing your body with vitality. With each exhale, release any lingering tension, allowing your body and mind to enter a state of serene receptivity.

This intentional act of breathing deeply serves as a gateway, harmonizing your being with the elements that await. As you approach the water, your senses attuned and your entire being calmed, you are poised to experience the profound connection between your breath, the water, and the vibrant life it sustains.

1. Emotional Resonance

As you approach the serene pond or flowing stream, be mindful of the emotions stirred within you by the presence of water. Let these emotions wrap around you, linking your soul with the deep reservoir of feelings experienced by every living being that embraces these waters.

How does the sound of flowing water affect your mood and state of mind?

Are there any memories or thoughts that arise as you stand near the water's edge?

2. Waterside Harmonies

Listen attentively as the water sings its soft, rhythmic melody. The gentle lapping against the shore, the occasional splash, and the rustle of leaves touched by droplets create a natural symphony. Allow these soothing sounds to envelop you, connecting you to the ancient rhythm of water, a fundamental life-force for all existence.

What observations can you make about the activities of wildlife, birds, insects, or frogs?

How does the proximity to the pond or stream impact your overall sense of wellbeing?

3. Aromatic Symphony

Engage your olfactory senses, embracing the subtle, earthy scent of water lingering in the air. Imagine it as a fragrant whisper, carrying the very essence of life. Let this aromatic dance enchant your senses, appreciating the intricate perfumes of nature.

Is there a distinct difference in the scent of the air?

How would you describe the scent of the air near the water?
What does it remind you of? Describe it as if you were tasting wine.

4. Dancing Light

Gaze upon the water's surface and witness the mesmerizing interplay of light and shadow. Observe as sunlight weaves ever-changing patterns, painting a canvas of colors and reflections. Witness the reflections of the surrounding trees and sky dancing on the water's surface, creating a mesmerizing tapestry of nature's artistry. Let this visual spectacle awaken your sense of wonder, immersing you in the peacefulness of the moment.

How does the movement of the water create patterns and shapes?

What patterns can you discern in the clouds? Does the water mirror the sky?

How does the sunlight filter through the branches, casting its glow on the Earth below?

5. Water's Serenity

Immerse yourself in the fluidity of water, observing its graceful movements and the melodic sounds it produces. Feel the gentle caress of water, grounding you in the present. Tune in to the soothing rhythm, harmonizing your being with nature's whispers that surround you.

How has this interaction with nature impacted your sense of presence and connection?

6. Submerged Secrets

Peer beneath the water's surface, exploring the hidden world beneath. Observe the diverse aquatic life and plants, each a testament to nature's intricate design. Witness the delicate balance of this underwater realm, appreciating the interconnectedness of all life forms beneath the surface with those above.

What lies beneath the surface that captures your curiosity?

Do you notice any interactions or behaviors among the underwater inhabitants that intrigue you? Explore the intricate interplay of nature's elements and lifeforms.

7. Landscapes Transformed

Contemplate the transformative influence of water on the surrounding environment. Reflect on its patient sculpting of valleys, nourishment of vegetation, and shaping of the Earth. Acknowledge the profound impact water wields, molding the landscape and enriching the very essence of the ecosystem.

Next time you take a refreshing sip of water, sense the water embracing its intrinsic purpose as it nourishes and becomes a vital presence within you, intimately connecting your essence with the natural world.

How does the importance of water's presence on Earth make you feel physically and emotionally?

Can you feel a sense of belonging as you witness the water's purposeful journey?

8. Tactile Connection

Find a comfortable spot by the water's edge, grounding yourself in the soft earth or smooth stones. Extend your hand, feeling the cool, refreshing touch of the water. Notice its texture, the way it caresses your skin, inviting you to fully immerse your senses. Imagine the stories it holds, the places it has traveled, and the life it has sustained.

What sensations arise as the water touches your skin?

What stories might the water be whispering to you as you touch it?

How does the touch of the water make you aware of your connection to the natural world?

Does this physical interaction with the water evoke any specific memories or thoughts?

9. Physical Immersion (Imagined or Real)

If allowed and safe, consider dipping your feet into the water. Feel the subtle ripples as they encircle your skin, embracing you in nature's gentle hug. Let the water's embrace remind you of the eternal cycle of renewal, encouraging you to release the past and embrace the endless possibilities that lie ahead.

How does the touch of the water make you aware of your connection to the natural world?

Can you sense the unity in this moment of tactile communion with water?

Does the feeling of the water change as you move your feet or hands?

What emotions or sensations arise as you connect with the water in this way?

10. Water's Essence

Inhale the serene atmosphere as you draw near the water, your senses awakened, and with each exhale, release any distractions, preparing to experience the profound interplay between your breath and the vibrant life nurtured by the water.

Open your senses to the gentle waves of resonance that flow through air, connecting you to the pulse of the universe. Water, the source of life, carries an ancient essence, flowing through the veins of the Earth. Allow yourself to attune to this vital essence, sensing the pulse of life in every ripple and wave. Connect with the timeless energy of water, understanding its role as a life-giving force that sustains not just your body, but also your soul. Feel the interconnectedness as you immerse yourself in the energy of the water's essence, absorbing the wisdom it holds. Let the energy of the water flow through you, harmonizing your own energy with the natural rhythms of the universe.

What emotions or insights arose as you tuned into the ancient essence surrounding the water?

Consider the impact of this experience on your overall wellbeing and spiritual connection.

Closing

After spending some moments in the soothing presence of water, find a quiet spot nearby to sit or stand. Take a few deep breaths, inhaling the calmness of the water, and exhale any remaining tension. In this sacred communion with water, express your profound gratitude for its life-sustaining essence and the unifying force it represents. Be thankful for the emotions it evokes, the beauty it unveils, and the intricate tapestry of life it nurtures. As you depart from this tranquil sanctuary, carry with you a deep sense of reverence for water's indispensable role in the intricate web of existence.

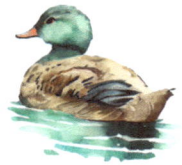

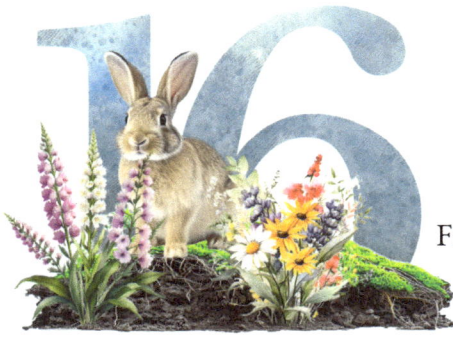

16 IMMERSING IN THE FRAGRANCE OF A FLOWER'S ESSENCE

Find a tranquil spot in nature, preferably near a blooming flower or tree. Sit or stand comfortably, grounding yourself in the natural environment. Close your eyes gently and take a few deep breaths. Inhale slowly, imagining you are drawing in the essence of the forest. As you exhale, release any tension or thoughts, allowing yourself to become fully present in this moment.

1. Embracing the Fragrance

Focus on the scent of the blooming flower. Inhale deeply, allowing its fragrance to fill your senses. Feel how the aroma gracefully caresses your skin and seeps into your very being. Let the fragrance surround you like a gentle, comforting embrace.

> Reflect on the potential for shared moments of sensory awareness to strengthen interpersonal bonds and foster a sense of unity with an-other.

2. Floral Symphony

Within the velvety folds of a flower's petals resides a harmonious blend of hundreds of chemical compounds, each contributing to the intricate orchestra of its floral essence.

Reach towards the flower and breathe slowly, taking 3 deliberate breaths. Inhale the sweet essence of the flower's fragrance, letting it infuse your breath, and as you exhale, allow the fragrant bloom to transport you to a serene state of mind.

Take a moment to explore this captivating composition. Envision the elegant interplay of molecules, each fulfilling a unique role in crafting the enchanting aroma. Reflect on the remarkable diversity and intelligence present in nature, savoring the meticulous balance that gives rise to these captivating scents. Within the delicate notes carried by flowers, there exists a unique olfactory signature—a finely tuned language that acts as a beacon, guiding the specific pollinator it beckons.

> How does it make you feel in the present moment?

Consider the intricate process through which plants produce these fragrances to attract pollinators. How does this natural mechanism inspire awe and appreciation for the intelligence of the natural world?

3. Contemplating the Flower's Purpose
Reflect on the reasons for the flower's existence. Consider how it evolved to produce this delicate, captivating scent. Contemplate the role of the flower in the ecosystem, attracting pollinators and adding beauty to the world.

What lessons might the flower hold about purpose and beauty?

4. The Eternal Essence
Once again, take another slow breath, allowing the delicate floral scent to fill your lungs, immersing yourself in its essence. Acknowledge that the fragrance of the flower, once experienced, becomes integrated into your body and memory, lingering within you forever.

Pause to recognize how this instant, entwined with the flower's scent, is etched into your soul, creating a timeless connection between you and nature.

5. The Cycle of Renewal
Reflect on the cyclical nature of the flower's life—its growth, bloom, and eventual withering away. Consider how this cycle mirrors the seasons of life, reminding you of the impermanence and the beauty in every stage of existence.

How does this natural cycle resonate with the different phases of your own life?

How does this awareness influence your perception of the present moment?

6. Integration of Fragrance and Memory
Contemplate how scents have a unique ability to trigger memories and emotions. Reflect on any memories or emotions that the fragrance of the flower has evoked.

How can you harness the power of scent in your daily life to create positive and meaningful experiences, or to evoke cherished memories?

Closing Reflection

Allow yourself to sit in this awareness for a moment longer, absorbing the essence of the flower's fragrance. When you're ready, gently open your eyes, feeling a renewed sense of connection to nature and a deeper understanding of the eternal, fleeting moments that shape our lives. The fragrance and gifts of this experience will be alive and carried somewhere within you forever. Allow it to inspire your journey and enrich your connection with the world around you.

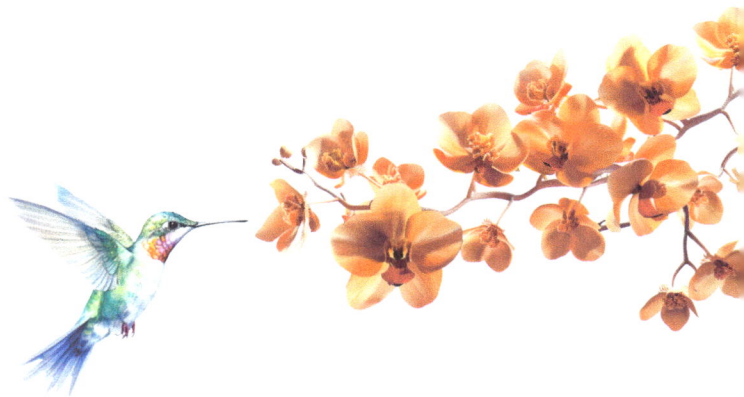

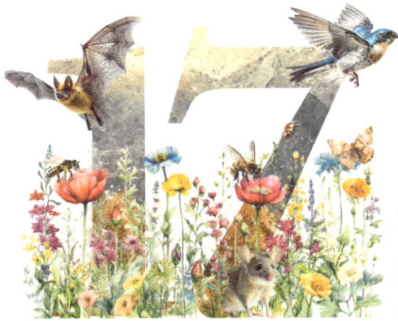

HONORING THE POLLINATORS' DANCE

In this nature experience, we step into the vibrant world of pollinators, the unsung heroes of nature. Embrace the fascinating dance of bees, butterflies, birds, bats, moths, flies, beetles, wasps, and even small mammals as they flit and hover around blossoms—every pollinator diligently performing their mission in the world.

Begin by taking a few deep breaths, grounding yourself in the present moment. Feel the subtle movements of nature around you and acknowledge the essential role of pollinators in this vibrant tapestry of life.

1. Observing Pollinator Activity

Find a tranquil spot amidst the blossoming flora, where the air is alive with the gentle hum of pollinators. Observe the pollinators in action, from bees to butterflies, bats to beetles. Notice the grace in their flight and the delicate way they collect nectar and pollen. Witness their importance in the pollination process, enabling plants to reproduce and thrive. Reflect on the beauty of their cooperation with the flora.

How do they move from flower to flower?

What colors are they attracted to?

How do the pollinators' movements make you feel?

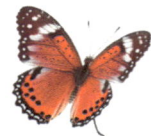

2. Connecting with Nature's Harmony

Close your eyes and tune in to the gentle hum of pollinators. Feel the vibrations of their wings in the air. Let their harmonious buzz resonate within you, a testament to nature's intricate symphony.

Acknowledge the unity between these creatures and the plants they serve. Contemplate the significance of this partnership in sustaining biodiversity.

How did embracing the buzz of pollinators impact your mind, body, and emotions?

Did you notice any changes in your thoughts, physical sensations, or emotional state?

3. Understanding Interconnectedness
Contemplate the ripple effect of pollinators' actions. Consider how their pollination efforts reverberate through the ecosystem, supporting not only plants but also animals and humans. Ponder on the delicate balance disrupted if their role were diminished. Embrace the realization of our interconnectedness, acknowledging the impact of these tiny beings on our daily lives.

> As you felt the interconnected threads binding you to these creatures, what emotions surfaced?

4. Reflecting on Conservation
Open your mind to the challenges faced by pollinators in the modern world. With each breath, acknowledge the complexities of their struggles and the delicate balance between their existence and the human-induced challenges these vital creatures endure.

Allow yourself to empathize deeply with the plight of pollinators. Feel their resilience amidst adversity, their determination to continue their vital work despite the odds stacked against them. Recognize the significance of their role in sustaining biodiversity and ensuring the pollination of countless plant species, including those we rely on for food.

> Reflect on your responsibility as a steward of nature. Consider how small changes in your lifestyle, like planting pollinator-friendly plants or supporting local organic farmers, can make a difference.

5. Immersing in Stillness
Sit in quiet contemplation, allowing the awareness of pollinators' importance to permeate your being. Feel the interconnected threads that bind you to these creatures and the natural world. Let a sense of responsibility and reverence grow within you. In this moment of stillness, pledge to protect and nurture the habitats that sustain pollinators.

> Reflect on the feelings of responsibility and reverence for pollinators that arose within you during this contemplative practice. How did these emotions manifest in your thoughts or body?

Closing

In the stillness of this moment, invite a profound sense of compassion to permeate your thoughts. Nurture the awareness of the importance that pollinators have in the world within your heart. Let it guide your actions and decisions, fostering a deeper respect for all beings that share this planet. As you step back into the world, remember the intricate dance of pollinators and cherish the vital role they play in the tapestry of life. Express your thanks silently or aloud, honoring their essential role in our world.

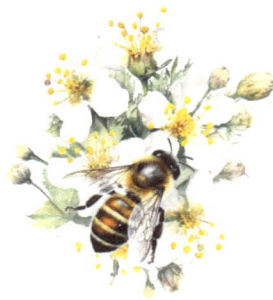

EMBRACING ANIMAL WISDOM

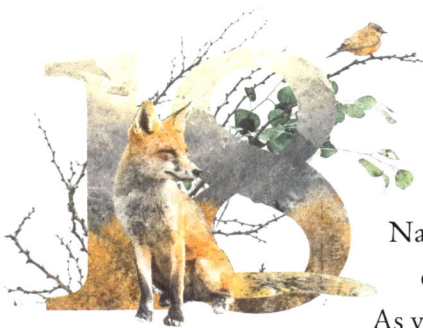

Nature's symphony invites you to become a part of its melody, embracing the marvels of existence that often go unnoticed. As you wander into the forest, consider it a sacred space, a home to diverse beings who share their world with you. Here, amid the tranquil embrace of nature, witness the subtle movements of animals. By quietly observing, explore their diverse personalities and the universal language they share with us. Through eyes unclouded by prejudice, appreciate their diverse intellect, recognizing the richness of their personalities. Each animal is a testament to nature's creativity, a unique individual with its own set of preferences, quirks, and emotions.

1. Breathing in Stillness

Inhale deeply, syncing your breath with the rhythm of the forest. As you exhale, release any tension, immersing yourself in the tranquility that surrounds you. In this state of stillness, witness the animals' unique personalities, appreciating their diverse expressions of life.

> Think about the diverse expressions of life displayed by the animals you observed. How do their unique personalities resonate with your own experiences and understanding of life?

> Reflect on the synchroneity of your breath with the forest's rhythm. How does this harmonious connection affect your sense of calm and presence in the moment?

2. Bonds and Expressions

Animals, much like humans, form bonds, express love, and nurture their young. Their playful frolics and joyous moments echo our own experiences, reminding you of the universal language of happiness. Witnessing their moments of tenderness and care, you appreciate the depth of their emotions, realizing the universality of love that binds all living beings.

> Contemplate the depth of emotions exhibited by the animals, recognizing the universality of love among all living beings. How does witnessing their emotional bonds broaden your perspective on the interconnectedness of life, and how can you nurture this awareness in your own interactions with the world?

Consider the universal language of happiness displayed by these animals. How does their joyous energy reflect the innate sense of happiness within yourself, and how can you draw inspiration from their playful frolics?

Reflect on the similarities between the animals' expressions of love and nurturing with your own experiences. How do these shared moments of tenderness resonate with your understanding of compassion and connection?

3. Contemplating Nature's Beauty

Occasionally, you observe animals gazing at the landscape, contemplating the beauty of nature. In those moments, you sense a profound connection between them and the environment, acknowledging their appreciation for the world's wonders. It serves as a reminder of the shared awe and reverence for life's mysteries, transcending the boundaries of species.

Reflect on the animals' contemplative moments as they gaze at the landscape. How does this shared appreciation dissolve the boundaries between species, highlighting the universal interconnectedness of all living beings?

In what ways can you cultivate a deeper connection with the natural world, mirroring their profound reverence?

4. Nature's Silent Conversations

Observe the animals, each engaged in their own world, yet united by the silent language of nature. In their individual pursuits, whether it's a bird building a nest, a squirrel foraging for food, or a deer grazing peacefully, they share an unspoken understanding with the environment around them. Notice the way their movements harmonize with the rhythms of the forest, blending seamlessly with the rustle of leaves, the gentle murmur of a stream, and the distant calls of fellow creatures. Witnessing this unity, you become attuned to the silent language that unites all living beings.

Consider the unspoken language shared between these animals and their surroundings. How does this silent communication reflect the deeper connections that exist within the natural world?

How might you cultivate a similar awareness in your interactions with others and your environment?

5. Bridging Hearts

Find a serene spot in the forest where you can comfortably observe the sky. Settle down on the soft earth or a cozy blanket, and let your gaze drift upward. Breathe in the crisp, fresh air of the forest, feeling it fill your lungs with rejuvenating energy. Turn your attention to a flock of birds gliding gracefully through the air above. Notice the seamless choreography of their flight, each bird instinctively synchronized with the others in a ballet of shared purpose. Reflect on this harmonious dance as a living testament to their bond, a large family brought together by an unwavering sense of belonging. Not one bird strays from the flock, and no one is left behind. Each wingbeat is a pledge of unity, each turn a promise of mutual trust. Breathe out, embracing the tranquil embrace of nature's rhythm, letting it wrap around you entirely. Feel the profound connection they share, a connection so deep and enduring it seems to pulse with the very heartbeat of the Earth. This connection is fueled by the natural life-force that underpins every yearning for companionship and unity, an elemental desire that transcends all Earthborn beings.

As you watch the flock of birds, their graceful coordination and mutual support become a symphony of togetherness. Their collective movement, effortless and elegant, whispers of ancient rhythms and the timeless dance of life. Let this avian ballet illuminate the beauty and strength found in togetherness, inspiring a deep sense of peace and harmony within you. Imagine yourself as part of this flock, moving through the world with the same grace and assurance, knowing that you, too, are never alone.

> In what ways does the concept of "togetherness" transcend species boundaries, uniting all living beings in a shared journey through life?
>
> What does belonging mean to you, and how does it influence your sense of self and purpose in the world?
>
> How do you personally cultivate and nurture the bonds of unity and trust within your community or family, drawing inspiration from the synchronized flight of birds?
>
> How do you see empathy playing a pivotal role in fostering understanding and cooperation among individuals, enabling us to move in harmony towards common objectives?

6. Contemplating Unity

As you witness animals gazing at the vast expanse of the forest, contemplate the unity that binds all living beings, transcending species and boundaries. Each creature, from the smallest insect to the majestic tree, plays a unique role in the symphony of existence. Contemplate the shared journey of growth, adaptation, and coexistence, recognizing the universal essence that unites all living entities.

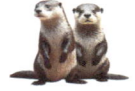

> How does witnessing the unity among animals in the forest inspire thoughts about your own interconnectedness with the world around you?

> Consider the challenges faced by different species in the forest and how they overcome them together. How can the unity observed among animals in nature serve as a lesson for human collaboration and coexistence?

7. Shared Consciousness

With every inhalation, recognize the invisible thread of shared consciousness that unites all living beings, weaving through the very fabric of existence. As you draw in the life-giving air, consider how this simple act connects you to every creature, every plant, and every being that breathes on this planet. Picture your breath mingling with the breath of ancient trees, with the whispers of the wind, and with the respiration of animals near and far. Inhale deeply, feeling the resonance of this shared life force within you.

> Consider the implications of a shared consciousness that transcends individuality. How might this understanding reshape your relationship with nature, animals, and fellow humans, fostering a profound sense of kinship and mutual understanding?

> Ponder the significance of breath as a life force. How does recognizing its shared nature deepen your understanding of the fundamental essence that unites all living things?

8. Witnessing Nature's Artistry

Take a moment to marvel at a spider web or a spider weaving its intricate web, crafting delicate silken threads strong enough to capture the fastest of insects. Observe the artistry in its creation, a testament to nature's precision and elegance. Reflect on the patience and skill required, finding inspiration in the spider's craftsmanship.

> Consider the artistry in the symphony of sounds, colors, and textures within a forest.

How can you cultivate a deeper connection to the natural world by recognizing it as an everchanging masterpiece, fostering a sense of awe and reverence for the creative artists and forces that shape our natural world?

Reflect on the interconnectedness of all life, observing how the spider's web sustains the balance of its ecosystem. How does this realization deepen your understanding of the symbiotic relationships in nature? How might it encourage you to nurture more harmonious connections within your own community and environment?

9. Embracing Cooperation

Shift your focus to the industrious ants working together, tirelessly carrying organic waste and contributing to the forest's cleanliness. Witness their collective effort, a reminder of the power of cooperation and collaboration in sustaining ecosystems. Acknowledge the importance of each small task in the grand tapestry of life.

Consider the knowledge possessed by animals, guiding them in tasks essential for their survival and to the balance of the ecosystem. How does this instinctual wisdom highlight the innate intelligence and intuition present in all creatures?

Explore the concept of reciprocity in the animal kingdom, where animals play vital roles in pollination, seed dispersal, and maintaining ecological balance. Reflect on the responsibilities humans have in reciprocating this balance. How can we ensure that our actions contribute positively to the wellbeing of animals and the environment, fostering a mutually beneficial relationship between humans and wildlife?

10. Symphony of Life

Listen to the gentle sway of flowers in the wind, a natural orchestra inviting bees to participate in the essential act of pollination. Observe the choreography of petals and the hum of bees, harmonizing to create fruits and seeds. Recognize the profound interconnectedness between flora and fauna, understanding the role each plays in sustaining life's vibrant cycle.

As you witness the inventiveness, skills, and craftsmanship in nature, what does your heart tell you about the profound creativity and resourcefulness inherent in all living beings?

Reflecting on the talents and artistry displayed by all living entities in nature, how does it evoke a profound appreciation for the ingenuity and cleverness that characterize all forms of life?

11. Embracing Diversity

In the heart of the forest, a vibrant tapestry of life unfolds, showcasing the extraordinary diversity of animals diligently contributing to the intricate balance of the ecosystem. Notice the harmonious collaboration among diverse animals flourishing, showcasing a unity untouched by discrimination or prejudice, reminding us of the beauty in genuine cooperation and acceptance across all species. Watch as squirrels dart between branches, gathering nuts for the winter, while industrious ants march in determined lines, efficiently recycling organic matter. Birds of myriad colors and melodies fill the air, pollinating flowers and dispersing seeds as they go. Beneath the canopy, a bustling community of insects toils, breaking down decaying matter into fertile soil. Each creature, from the tiniest beetle to the majestic bear, plays a unique role, ensuring the smooth functioning of nature's ecosystem. Recognizing this diversity not only deepens our understanding of nature's complexity but also fosters a profound respect for the harmonious collaboration that allows all life to flourish.

> How does awe manifest in your body and mind when you witness animals contributing to the vibrant orchestra of existence, united by the silent language of nature?

> Reflect on the sense of purpose animals demonstrate in their roles within the forest. How can you embody a similar sense of purpose in your daily activities and contributions to the world?

> Consider the lessons of unity and acceptance observed in the collaborative efforts of various animals. How can these lessons be applied to human interactions and societal harmony, promoting understanding and cooperation among people from diverse backgrounds?

Closing Reflection

Breathe deeply, grounding yourself in the stillness of the forest. In this quiet moment, express gratitude for the diverse forms of life surrounding you. Each being, from the towering trees to the tiniest insects, pave the way for the flourishing of all life forms.

Appreciate the wisdom and grace displayed by every creature, each contributing its unique essence to the intricate masterpiece of life. Bask in the splendor of this harmonious existence, and express deep thanks for the invaluable lessons learned and the awe-inspiring beauty witnessed. With profound appreciation, offer gratitude for the diverse and intelligent wonders of the natural world, forever inspiring you with their brilliance.

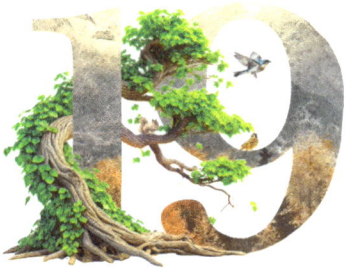

SENSING THE ELEMENTAL ESSENCE OF THE WIND

Find a peaceful spot in nature where you can comfortably sit or stand. Close your eyes and allow yourself to relax and be fully present in the moment. Inhale deeply, feeling the untamed essence of the wind, letting it intertwine with your breath, and as you exhale, release any stagnant energy, becoming one with the invisible dance of air that surrounds you.

Feel the ground beneath you, connecting with the Earth, and then shift your focus to the subtle yet profound presence of the wind around you. Allow yourself to sit in this awareness for a moment longer, absorbing the elemental essence of the wind.

1. Feel the Caress of the Wind

Open your palms and arms, inviting the wind to gently touch your skin. Feel its soft, cool or warm embrace as it wraps around you. Notice how it moves, dances, and plays with your senses. Embrace the sensation as the wind tenderly caresses your face and body.

> How does the sensation of the wind on your skin make you aware of your own physical presence in the moment?

> Reflect on a moment when you felt particularly attuned to the wind. What insights or revelations did you experience during that moment of connection?

2. Embracing Air's Sensations

Observe whether the air feels humid, dry, chilly, or warm against your skin. Notice how each of these sensations carries a unique energy, shaping the way you experience the moment. Inhale deeply, feeling the subtle variations in temperature and moisture, allowing your senses to attune to the subtle changes in the atmosphere. Let these sensations remind you of the ever-shifting nature of the world around you, inviting you to be fully present in this moment. Pause to acknowledge the air's adaptability, how it can provide refreshment on a scorching day, exhibit strength amidst a storm, bring invigoration on a crisp evening, or offer solace in its tender caress.

How does the wind's ability to both calm and intensify evoke the range of emotions within you? Reflect on the different emotional states the wind may represent for you.

3. Taste the Essence of the Air

Inhale deeply, tasting the freshness of the wind as it enters your lungs. Notice any scents or fragrances carried by the wind. Feel the purity of the air as it fills you, energizing your body and mind. Let the taste of the wind awaken your senses.

Reflect on the contrast between the purity of the air and the complexities of daily life. How does this awareness impact your perspective on simplicity and nature's elegance?

4. Smell the Aroma of Nature

As the wind carries various scents from the surrounding environment, identify the subtle fragrances it brings to you. Whether it's the aroma of blooming flowers, earthy soil, or distant rain, breathe in deeply and allow these natural scents to envelop you, creating a harmonious symphony of smells.

Which of the scents carried by the wind resonates with you the most, and why do you think it has a particular impact on your senses?

How do these natural fragrances symbolize the interconnectedness of all living things, and what can we learn from this harmonious symphony of smells?

5. Touch of Connection

Extend your hand towards the wind and gently touch it with your fingertips. Feel its intangible yet powerful presence against your skin. Notice how it moves through your fingers. Sense the energy and vitality it carries within its intangible form. Can you find a sense of freedom in the wind's boundless movement?

How does this freedom resonate with your own desires for liberation and exploration?

6. The Purpose of the Wind

Ponder on the purpose of the wind in nature. Consider how it disperses seeds, carries essential nutrients, and maintains the balance of ecosystems. Reflect on its role in shaping the environment and supporting life.

How might the wind's purpose resonate with your own purpose in life?

7. Understanding the Wind's Journey

Contemplate the wind's journey, realizing that it travels across vast distances, touching various landscapes and people before touching you. Imagine the stories it carries from distant lands and diverse cultures. Reflect on the shared experiences it carries, connecting humanity in ways we may not always perceive.

Contemplate the idea of the wind touching others before reaching you. How does this interconnectedness make you feel?

What insights does it offer about the shared experiences of humanity?

Closing

In the soft whispers of the wind, you find gratitude for its invisible touch, a reminder of the intangible yet profound connections that bind you to the natural world. As you breathe in its whispers, you are grateful for the life it carries, the secrets it shares, and the dances it orchestrates through the leaves. May you always be attuned to the songs of the wind, acknowledging its presence as a constant companion on your journey through this beautiful, interconnected world

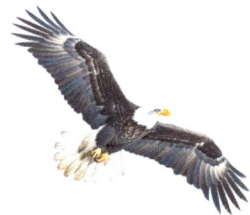

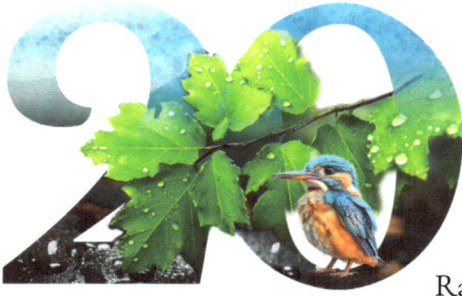

RAIN'S TENDER TOUCH

In the tranquil heart of the forest, allow yourself to be caressed by the soothing touch of raindrops. Rain, the Earth's gentle healer, whispers stories of life as it dances upon leaves and soil. Embrace this natural symphony, connecting deeply with the life-giving essence of the rain.

1. Inviting Rain's Arrival
Find a serene spot amidst the trees. Close your eyes and stand with arms outstretched, palms turned upward, inviting the rain to grace your skin. Feel the first droplets kiss your face and hands, acknowledging the arrival of this life-giving elixir.

How does the initial touch of rain make you feel?

2. Engaging Your Senses
Tune in to the sounds of raindrops drumming on leaves, rocks, and the forest floor. Let the melody of rain serenade your ears. Notice the scent of wet earth rising, mingling with the forest's natural aroma.

How does the aroma of rain differ from the forest's usual scent?

How did the sound of raindrops and the scent of wet earth affect your mood during the experience?

3. Dancing with Raindrops
Take a leisurely stroll, allowing raindrops to caress your skin. Feel the cool, refreshing touch of water droplets. Observe how they cling to leaves and petals, reflecting the surrounding world in miniature.

How does the sensation of raindrops on your skin awaken your senses?

4. Rain's Melodic Harmony
Find shelter under a tree and listen to the symphony of raindrops composing melodies as

they patter on different surfaces. For a few moments, close your eyes, and let the gentle patter of raindrops weave a timeless thread, connecting your heart to the timeless heartbeat of nature.

How do these raindrop rhythms resonate within you?

Do they evoke specific emotions or memories?

Consider the symphony of raindrops on various surfaces. Did it inspire any creative thoughts or emotions within you?

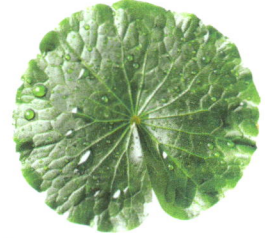

5. Communing with Nature

Observe how the rain rejuvenates the forest, invigorating colors and scents. The colors seem to deepen, and the scents intensify, as if nature itself is taking a deep breath. Each raindrop, a precious elixir, revives the Earth, reminding us of the delicate balance that sustains life in the forest.

How does this natural revival inspire you?

Can you sense the interconnectedness between the rain, the forest, and your own existence?

6. Embracing the Rain's Blessing

Stand in the rain, arms outstretched, and allow it to imaginally cleanse your entire being. Feel the raindrops merging with your essence, washing away any worries or tensions. With each droplet, a sense of renewal permeates your being, connecting you deeply to the Earth's rhythm. Let the rain be a reminder of your resilience, just like the forest embracing the storm, finding strength in vulnerability.

How does this cleansing ritual affect your mood and mindset?

How do you perceive the world after this moment of renewal?

Closing

In the soft caress of raindrops, we discover the whisper of ancient rhythms, a melody played by the universe. As you rejoin the world, remember the subtle symphony of the rain, its tender touch, and the sweet scent that lingers. Carry this moment with you, a reminder of your seamless connection with the natural tapestry. Whenever rain graces the Earth, let this memory be your refuge, grounding you in the essence of life's cycles. May the memory of this rain's embrace guide you back to nature's heart, offering solace and serenity whenever you seek refuge in its embrace.

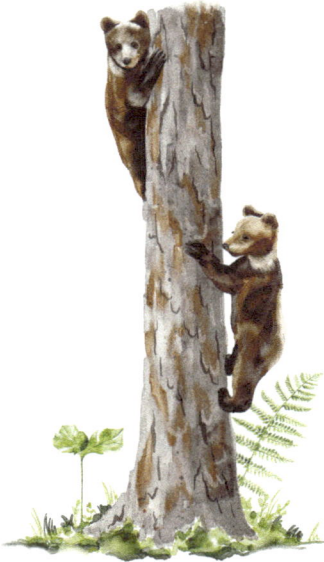

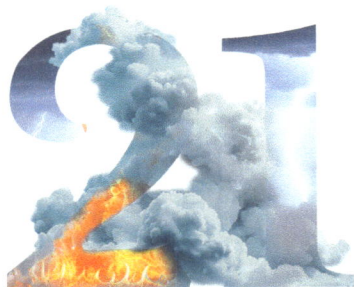

THE ELEMENTAL DANCE OF FIRE, THUNDER, AND LIGHTNING

In this nature therapy practice, you engage the primal elements of fire, thunder, and lightning. These forces of nature have long held a profound significance, symbolizing both destruction and illumination. Immerse yourself in their symbolic richness and engage in practices that connect you deeply with these elemental energies.

As you inhale, imaginally draw in the essence of fire, feeling its transformative power within you. As you exhale, release any stagnation or negativity, allowing fire's energy to cleanse and renew.

1. Connecting with Fire's Essence

Begin by envisioning a roaring bonfire or a single, flickering candle flame. Feel the warmth and energy it emits, symbolizing the essence of fire. Imagine yourself surrounded by its protective glow, acknowledging its role as a mediator between forms, transforming and transmuting all things.

> How does the flickering flame make you feel, embodying the dual nature of fire as both creator and destroyer?

> Hold your hands over an imaginary flame. Feel the warmth and visualize it transmuting any negative energy into positive, vibrant light within you.

2. Invoking Life

Visualize a stormy sky, heavy with dark clouds gathering above like an ancient congregation. With each roll of thunder, imagine it as the celestial orchestra heralding life-giving rain. Envision the raindrops descending gracefully, touching the Earth with gentle yet purposeful caresses, symbolizing not just renewal but a profound cleansing of the land. Picture the parched soil eagerly absorbing this liquid gift, awakening dormant seeds and breathing life into the landscape. In this imagery, find the harmony of nature's cycles, where storms are not just disruptions but transformative acts of rejuvenation, reminding you of the beauty in both chaos and rebirth.

Envision yourself standing in the gentle rain, letting it cleanse your being, washing away any doubts or fears, and leaving you with a pure and rejuvenated soul.

3. Embracing Thunder's Echoes

Close your eyes and listen to the echoes of thunder resonating through the atmosphere. Allow the sound to wash over you. Embrace the echoes of thunder as a reminder of nature's rhythm, the dualism of life, and its ability to embrace both good and bad, recognizing them as integral parts of existence. With each echo, feel a sense of acceptance and inner peace, knowing that life's challenges are opportunities for growth.

> Sit or stand in a comfortable position and close your eyes. Focus on the sound of thunder, feeling its vibrations within your body. As you breathe, let go of any resistance and accept the rhythm of life.

> How does the sound of thunder resonate within you, embodying the cycle of renewal and transformation?

4. Lightning's Illumination

Envision a lightning bolt streaking across the sky, illuminating the darkness with its sudden brilliance. Reflect on lightning as a symbol of sudden illumination, representing the destruction of ignorance and the revelation of hidden truths. Allow its energy to spark inspiration within you.

> How does the image of lightning resonate with your own moments of sudden insight and enlightenment?

5. Solar Connection

Picture the sun as the ultimate source of energy, radiating its light and warmth. Imagine a ray of lightning descending from the sun, carrying a creative force, a skilled architect, adept in shaping and upholding the material essence of the universe. Feel this energy merging with your being, igniting your creativity and illuminating your path.

> Stand in sunlight, with your arms outstretched, absorbing the sun's energy. Imagine a golden ray of lightning entering your body, infusing you with creativity and purpose.

6. Life's Stirring Awakening

Embrace the vibrant dance of flames as they flicker and leap, illuminating the darkness with their mesmerizing glow. Feel the warmth emanating from the fire, a life-giving force that has fueled human existence for millennia. Imagine the ancient rituals and stories carried in the crackling embers, connecting you to the profound wisdom of your ancestors. As you gaze into the heart of the fire, recognize its ability to stimulate life and inspire passion, provide heat and nourishing food, and to foster community. Let the flickering flames remind you of the resilience of life, embracing the dualism of human life, both good and bad, as part of your journey.

> As you feel the warmth of the flames caressing your skin, how does your body respond? Notice any sensations, tingling, or relaxation that arises, connecting you to the vitality of fire.

> With each flicker and dance of the flames, how does your breath synchronize? Pay attention to the rhythm of your breathing as it mirrors the mesmerizing movements of the fire, deepening your connection to the element's energy.

> As you absorb the radiant heat, envision it revitalizing your body's cells, bringing a renewed sense of energy and passion. How does this warmth manifest within you? Can you feel the rejuvenating power of fire awakening your senses and invigorating your being?

7. Bathing in the Elemental Dance

Imagine yourself surrounded by the crackling energy of fire, the echoing voices of thunder, and the illuminating flashes of lightning. Feel the primal forces intertwining around you, embracing both the destructive and transformative aspects of existence. Embrace the feeling of being a part of this elemental dance, connected to the ancient wisdom embedded within these natural phenomena.

> How does it feel to be in the midst of this elemental dance, symbolizing the eternal cycle of creation, destruction, and rebirth?

> Feel the warmth of the fire on your skin. Imagine it purifying not just your surroundings but also your mind and body.

Closing Reflection

As you move forward in the world, carry the energy of fire, thunder, and lightning within you. Express deep gratitude for their powerful energy that has enveloped you. Acknowledge their presence in your life, embracing the dualism they represent, reminding you of the balance between light and shadow, good and bad. Just as these elemental forces shape the natural world, they also shape your own journey of growth and transformation. Carry their wisdom with you, allowing them to illuminate you on your path and inspire your steps forward.

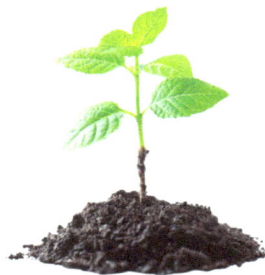

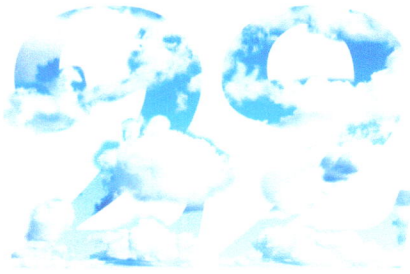

SKYWARD EMBRACE

As you step into the heart of nature, find a serene spot in the surrounding landscape where the open sky stretches endlessly above you. Feel the Earth beneath you, grounding your presence. Inhale deeply, drawing in the crisp, invigorating air of the outdoors, filling your lungs with the essence of nature's breath. As you exhale slowly, release any tension or limitations, allowing them to dissipate into the atmosphere like wisps of cloud. Feel the weight of the world lifting off your shoulders with each breath, surrendering to the infinite universe beyond.

Let your gaze rise above, toward the vast expanse of the sky. The sky, a canvas painted with everchanging hues, holds many secrets of the universe. Immerse yourself in the celestial wonders above, connecting with the boundless sky, the drifting clouds, and the radiant sun.

Find a comfortable spot, whether sitting or standing, where the open sky is in full view. Gently tilt your head upward and let your eyes roam the infinite heavens. Notice the expanse, the shades of blue, the interplay of light and shadow. Embrace the sense of vastness that the sky offers. Allow your awareness to expand as you acknowledge the endless possibilities stretching out before you.

1. Echoes of the Cosmos

Consider, in the tapestry of eternity, you're not merely a spectator, but a radiant presence woven into the universe's intricate dance. Your essence mirrors the vast expanse of the sky, the fiery brilliance of the sun, the gentle allure of the moon, and the twinkling constellations of stars. Embrace your role as a celestial being, for within you resides the eternal essence that unites all things in the cosmic symphony of existence.

Describe your presence within the tapestry of eternity.

2. Dancing Clouds

Observe the clouds, those ethereal wanderers adrift in the sky. Watch as they drift lazily or race hurriedly across the sky. Observe their formations—soft and billowy, wispy and delicate, or thick and dramatic. Notice how they cast shadows on the landscape below, creating a dance of light and darkness. Let your imagination roam, finding familiar shapes or creatures within their shifting forms.

> How did observing the sky and clouds make you feel? Did any of these forms resonate with you in a particular way?

3. Solar Connection

Feel the warmth of the sun on your skin, the source of life that illuminates the world. Observe the play of light and shadow as the sun moves across the sky, painting a masterpiece that shifts and evolves with each passing moment. Close your eyes and turn your face toward the sun. Feel its gentle caress and acknowledge its vital energy. Imagine the sun's rays permeating your being, filling you with light and positivity.

> How did the warmth of the sun affect your mood and energy?
> Did it bring a sense of vitality or relaxation?

4. Connect with the Moon's Glow

If the moon graces the sky, let your gaze be drawn towards its gentle radiance. Contemplate the moon's phases—whether it's a waxing crescent, a full moon illuminating the night, or a waning crescent slowly fading away. Consider the stories and myths that cultures around the world have woven around the moon. Reflect on how its serene presence has inspired poets, lovers, and dreamers throughout time.

> Does gazing at the moon stir particular emotions or memories within you? Can you identify the bodily sensations associated with these emotions?

5. Feel the Openness

Allow the vastness of the sky to fill your awareness. Imagine your being expanding, reaching out towards the celestial dome above you. Feel the vastness in your heart and mind as you acknowledge your presence in this infinite universe, which includes up to two trillion galaxies in the observable universe. Recognize that, like the sky, sun, moon, and stars, you are a part of something grand and eternal.

> In what ways do you feel interconnected with the sky, clouds, sun, and the boundless cosmos?

> As you acknowledge this immense cosmic expanse, bring your attention to your heart center.

Can you sense the energy of the universe resonating within you? How does this connection with universal energy manifest physically, perhaps as warmth, tingling, or a sense of expansion?

Imagine your mind expanding to encompass the vast universe, realizing the limitless possibilities that exist within this boundless space. Picture your thoughts reaching out into the cosmic expanse, touching the mysteries of distant galaxies. How does this awareness of your presence in the infinite universe make you feel within your body and soul?

6. Celestial Symphony

Listen to the sounds of the sky. Hear the rustle of leaves as the wind passes through, the distant calls of birds soaring high above, and the gentle whispers of the breeze. Connect with these sounds, allowing them to harmonize with the rhythm of your own breath. Feel the symphony of nature enveloping you, a melody composed by the elements.

Which sounds from the sky resonated with you the most? How did they enhance your experience of nature's symphony?

7. Nightfall Wonder

Close your eyes. Imagine the night sky, a canvas sprinkled with stars, each one a distant sun in its own right. Picture the constellations, the moonlight casting a soft glow upon the world. Envision the sense of mystery and awe that comes with the night. Embrace the quiet beauty of the nocturnal world, where the sky becomes a tapestry of dreams and aspirations.

As you imagined the night sky, what emotions or thoughts arose? Did it evoke a sense of wonder or contemplation about the universe?

Closing

Express gratitude for this moment of connection with the heavenly bodies above. Acknowledge the wonder and awe they inspire within you. Be thankful for the perspective they offer, reminding you of the boundless beauty of the cosmos. Reflect on the vastness of the universe and your place within it. Consider how this experience has widened your perspective and brought a sense of peace and unity. As you lower your gaze, let this awareness of the infinite beauty above you nurture your soul, providing a gentle reminder of the interconnectedness of all things in this vast cosmic dance. Inhale deeply once more, absorbing the energy of the sky, and as you exhale, release your gratitude into the universe.

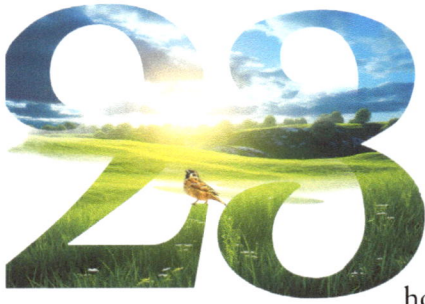

SUNRISE SERENITY

Choose a spot in the forest where you can fully appreciate the grandeur of the sunrise. Ideally, this should be a location with an unobstructed view of the eastern horizon. As you settle into your chosen position, whether it be on a natural rock formation, a fallen log, or a patch of soft moss, ensure that you have a clear and expansive view of the sky.

Allow your body to relax, grounding yourself in the natural surroundings. Close your eyes and take a few deep breaths. Inhale deeply, feeling the crisp morning air fill your lungs, and exhale slowly, releasing any tension. Repeat this mindful breathing, syncing your breath with the rhythm of nature.

1. Sunrise Gazing

As the sun makes its ascent, open your eyes slowly to witness the magic of the sunrise. At first, the sky and clouds may be painted in subtle hues of pink, lavender, and orange. Focus your gaze on the changing colors, observing the gradual transformation of the sky from the darkness of night to the brilliance of day.

Take note of the interplay between light and shadow among the trees. The early morning sunlight filters through the leaves, casting intricate patterns on the forest floor. Notice how the branches and leaves absorb and reflect the golden hues, creating a dance of light that is unique to this moment.

Allow your eyes to follow the sun's journey as it rises above the horizon. Observe the way the landscape is gradually illuminated, unveiling the details of the forest that were concealed in the predawn darkness. Take in the silhouette of the trees against the brightening sky, appreciating the contrast between the stillness of the night and the awakening of a new day.

As you gaze at the sunrise, be present in the moment. Resist the urge to capture it through a lens; instead, imprint the beauty of the scene in your mind. Feel the warmth of the sunlight on your face and the gentle caress of the morning breeze. Let the serenity of the forest envelop you, creating a connection between the natural world and your own inner peace.

In this simple act of sunrise gazing, you become a silent observer of nature's daily masterpiece, acknowledging the cyclical rhythm of the Earth and the beauty that unfolds with each new dawn.

> Consider the ephemeral nature of the sunrise, how it marks the beginning of a new day and the passage of time. How does the sunrise inspire you to embrace the present and appreciate the beauty in each passing moment?

> Take notice of the serene atmosphere that often accompanies the sunrise. Embody the stillness by becoming aware of your own body's posture and movements. How does the stillness of the forest and the tranquil dawn affect your own sense of presence? What physical sensations arise as you allow the calmness of the morning to settle within you?

> As you gaze at the rising sun, focus on the warmth it imparts to the surroundings. Tune into the physical sensations in your own body. Where do you feel warmth or a subtle energy awakening within you? How does the sensation of warmth embody a connection between the external natural world and your internal physical experience?

2. Invitation for World Healing

Inhale gently, attuning your ears to the melodic symphony of birdsongs, and with each exhale, let go of the noise of the world, allowing the soothing notes to guide you into a meditative dance with our feathered Earthborn companions.

In the ancient echoes of a time long past, a profound wisdom resonates—the belief that the songs at dawn and songs at dusk possess the transformative power to heal the world with beauty. Entrusted to the custodianship of the birds, these keepers of forgotten lore remind us each morning with their songs that the world is inherently meant for joy and peace. Embrace this new day, drawing forth the melodies within your heart to heal the world and sow the seeds of peace on Earth. Encourage the enchanting notes of peace to ripple across the vast expanse of the Earth, and, in this collective harmony, as you breathe in the serenity of nature, let every exhale be a gentle release, sending gentle waves of unity and harmony into the world from the depths of your heart.

In what ways does your breath synchronize with the songs of the birds at dawn, fostering an embodied experience of peacefulness and the belief in the inherent peace of the world?

As you embrace the new day and encourage the enchanting notes of peace to ripple across the Earth, explore how this intention resonates within your physical body. How do sensations, perhaps in your chest or breath, reflect your embodied commitment to healing and sowing the seeds of peace on Earth?

Closing

Sit or stand with a sense of stillness, and close your eyes for a brief moment to internalize the beauty you've just witnessed. Feel the warmth of the emerging sun on your skin, and take a few intentional breaths, inhaling the invigorating scent of the forest.

As you open your eyes and the sun rises higher in the sky, take a moment to reflect on the beauty of the experience. Express gratitude for the tranquility, the beauty of nature, and the opportunity to witness the sunrise in the company of the forest.

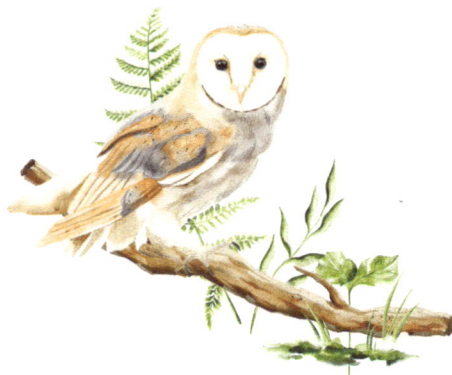

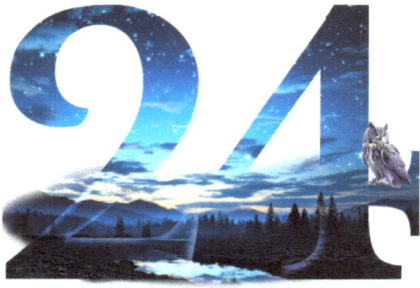

SUNSET'S TRANQUIL TWILIGHT

Position yourself strategically within the heart of the forest, ensuring an unobstructed view of the western horizon. This carefully chosen vantage point allows you to fully immerse yourself in the enchanting spectacle about to unfold. Take a moment to stand or sit comfortably, attuning your senses to the ambient sounds of the forest, the cool embrace of the air, and the anticipation that lingers in the quietude.

Begin by breathing in the soothing essence of the approaching sunset through your nose, allowing the tranquil energy to fill your lungs. Hold this serene breath briefly, immersing yourself in the calming atmosphere. As you exhale slowly through your mouth, release any lingering tension, and imagine exhaling out the stresses of the day. With each breath, envision becoming one with the rhythmic heartbeat of the forest, syncing your breath to the gentle cadence of the twilight hour.

1. Twilight Meditation

As the sun embarks on its descent, let your gaze be drawn towards the horizon. The initial warmth of the sunlight paints the sky in a palette of soft oranges, pinks, and golds, casting a warm glow over the landscape. Fix your eyes on the evolving canvas above, noticing the subtle dance of clouds catching the last rays of the day.

Observe the seamless transition of colors as the sun inches lower, signaling the gradual shift from the warmth of daylight to the cool, calming tones of dusk. The sky transforms into a canvas of purples, blues, and grays, creating a serene backdrop against the silhouette of the trees. The forest, once bathed in brilliant daylight, now takes on a dreamlike quality as shadows lengthen and branches become intricate lace against the fading light.

Take a moment to appreciate the reflections of sunlight on leaves, turning the forest into a living kaleidoscope. The foliage becomes a canvas for the intricate patterns of light and shadow, each leaf capturing the essence of the waning sunlight. This visual symphony unfolds around you, a harmonious collaboration between nature's elements.

Feel the lingering warmth on your skin as the sun makes its final descent. The sunlight becomes a gentle caress, a fleeting connection between the celestial sphere and the earthly realm. In this dimming light, become aware of the delicate sounds of the forest, a prelude to the nocturnal chorus that will soon begin.

As the sun disappears below the horizon, embrace the gradual dimming of the forest. The transition from daylight to twilight is a metaphor for the ebb and flow of life, a poignant reminder of the beauty found in transitions and the acceptance of the inevitable cycles of change. In this sacred moment of sunset gazing, surrender to the beauty of the natural world's farewell to the day. Let the interplay of warm and cool colors, the reflection of sunlight on leaves, and the gradual dimming of the forest become a meditation on the ephemeral nature of existence and the timeless beauty that emerges in the twilight hours. Allow the enchantment of the sunset to linger in your senses as you bid farewell to the day, finding solace in the serene embrace of the evening forest.

> How does the act of observing the sunset foster a connection between the vastness of the universe and your own sense of purpose and meaning? Ponder the cosmic perspective offered by the sunset, contemplating the sheer magnitude of the universe against the backdrop of your own experiences. Consider how this celestial event encourages introspection about your place in the grand tapestry of existence and the pursuit of personal purpose and fulfillment.

> How does the sensation of the cooling evening air against your skin contribute to your embodied experience of the sunset? Explore the tactile elements of the sunset experience, considering the temperature changes, the gentle caress of the breeze, and how these sensations ground you in the present moment.

> In what ways does your body respond to the diminishing light and the emerging shadows during the sunset? Pay attention to the physical reactions and subtle movements within your body as the sunlight fades. Notice changes in posture, muscle tension, or even the way your senses heighten in the dimming light, enhancing your embodied connection to the evolving atmosphere.

2. Nature's Nighttime Soundscape

Close your eyes and allow your ears to become the primary receptors of the surrounding world. Embrace the symphony of the night as it unfolds—a chorus of frogs with their rhythmic croaks, the enchanting melody of crickets creating a harmonious background, and the occasional rustle of leaves in the gentle breeze. Feel the cool touch of the wind brushing against your skin, becoming a subtle yet integral part of the nocturnal orchestra. Absorb the diverse soundscape, tuning into the unique voices of the nocturnal creatures and the soothing whispers of the wind. Let each sound become a thread in the tapestry of the evening, weaving a story of life in the darkness. Inhale the earthy scents carried by the wind, exhaling any lingering tension. With each breath, sink deeper into the tranquility of the night, allowing the vibrant sounds of nature, accompanied by the gentle wind, to envelop you in a comforting serenade. As you listen to the night's orchestration, let the wind become a gentle guide, connecting you to the natural rhythm and serenity of the nocturnal world.

> Explore the resonance of the nocturnal sounds within your chest and body. How do these vibrations deepen your connection to the natural orchestra, allowing you to feel the pulsating life of the forest during the night?

> Consider the role of the wind in shaping the auditory landscape of the night. How does the wind's subtle or forceful presence contribute to the overall embodied experience, guiding your attention and influencing the rhythm of your breath in this tranquil nocturnal setting?

Closing

In the hushed moments as the last rays of sunlight bid farewell, express gratitude for the ephemeral beauty that unfolded before you. Inhale deeply, drawing in the essence of renewal and transition that the sunset represents. Sense the stillness and promise of the approaching night. As you exhale, release anything that no longer serves you, letting it dissolve into the fading light. Thank the sun for painting the sky with its vibrant hues, the forest for sharing its quiet wisdom, and the tranquil evening for wrapping you in a blanket of peace. As you carry the calmness of the dusk within, be thankful for the beauty witnessed and the peace cultivated in this sacred twilight.

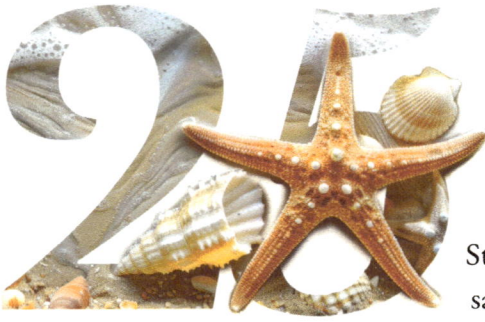

25 EMBRACING THE TRANQUILITY OF THE OCEAN

Stand at the edge of the ocean shore. Breathe in the salty sea air, filling your lungs with its rejuvenating essence, feeling it weave calm into your soul. The rhythmic waves whisper ancient tales, and the salty breeze gently caresses your skin. Let the ocean's melody guide you into a serene realm where nature's harmony meets the endless horizon. Embrace the therapeutic power of the sea and allow it to rejuvenate your senses. As you breathe out, immerse yourself fully in the calming embrace of the ocean, releasing tension and worries to the rhythm of the sea.

Now picture yourself floating on the water, weightless and free. The ocean cradles you, its currents intertwining with the breath of all life, linking you to the heartbeat of the Earth. Every wave, every ripple, echoes the pulse of life, from the tiniest sea creatures to the vast forests beyond. Drift in this serene, intimate space, feeling the profound connection that unites all living beings. Carry this tranquility within you as you step into today.

1. Arrival at the Shore
Stand at the water's edge. Close your eyes and take deep, calming breaths, allowing the salty aroma to fill your lungs. Feel the sand beneath your feet and the cool, refreshing touch of the ocean waves. With each step, be mindful of the sensations—the temperature, the texture of the sand beneath the water, and the subtle shifts in the waves. Engage all your senses in this immersive experience.

> How do the sensations of the sand beneath your feet and the cool touch of the ocean waves affect your body?

> As you breathe in the salty aroma of the ocean, how does it make you feel? Does it evoke any memories or emotions?

2. Breathing with the Tide
With each inhalation, visualize the tide pulling in, filling you with tranquility and energy.

As you exhale, imagine the tide retreating, carrying away any tension or negativity. Sync your breath with the natural ebb and flow of the ocean.

> How does the visualization of the tide pulling in and filling you with tranquility manifest in your body? Are there physical sensations or areas of your body where you feel this tranquility most profoundly?

> As you exhale and visualize the tide retreating, carrying away tension, how does this mental imagery influence your physical state? Notice any changes in muscle tension, heart rate, or overall relaxation as you sync your breath with the ocean's rhythm.

3. Listening to the Symphony

Tune in to the soothing melody of the ocean. Listen to the waves crashing against the shore, the seagulls' distant calls, and the rustling of the coastal trees and seagrasses. Let these sounds wash over you, immersing yourself in the symphony of the sea.

> What emotions or sensations do these sounds evoke within you?

> How does this auditory experience connect you to the essence of the ocean?

> Consider the different sounds of the ocean, each carrying its own energy and rhythm. Which sound resonates with you the most, and why?

4. Visualizing the Deep Blue

Close your eyes and visualize the vastness of the ocean, its deep blue expanse stretching infinitely. Imagine the life teeming beneath the surface—colorful fish, graceful dolphins, and majestic whales. Envision their movements, hear their voices, and sense the interconnectedness of all life forms.

> As you visualize the diverse marine life, how does their presence make you feel?

> As you imagine the voices of dolphins and whales, what emotions do these sounds evoke? How does this emotional response reflect your deep connection to the ocean and its inhabitants?

5. Communing with Marine Life

Take a moment to observe the underwater world, teeming with colorful fish darting among coral reefs. Witness their synchronized movements, showcasing the harmony of their community. Reflect on the vital roles these fish play in the ecosystem—from maintaining coral health to controlling algae levels.

Feel a sense of kinship with these creatures. Consider how their shared purpose, unity, and collaboration contributes to the ocean's balance, fostering a habitat where diverse species thrive.

> Feel a sense of kinship with the underwater creatures, acknowledging their presence as fellow beings on this planet. Engage in a gentle, flowing movement, mimicking the fluidity of their underwater dance. Notice how your body's motions evoke a profound connection, bridging the gap between species.

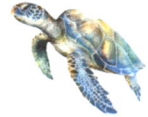

6. Appreciating Nature's Wisdom

Observe how sea plants sway with the rhythm of the currents, their adaptive features allowing them to thrive in the dynamic and challenging underwater environment. As you witness these phenomena, acknowledge the complexity of marine life, each species playing a vital role in the intricate web of life beneath the ocean's surface—all of this unfolding beyond our sight.

> How does acknowledging the existence of this hidden realm inspire your curiosity about the unknown aspects of life? Reflect on how embracing the unseen can broaden your perspective on the world around you.

> Contemplate the emotions stirred within you when thinking about the unseen wonders beneath the ocean. Is it awe, excitement, or perhaps a sense of humility? How do these emotions shape your understanding of the mysteries that exist beyond our sight?

> Imagine yourself diving into the depths of the ocean, exploring the unseen world with every stroke. How does this imaginal journey make you feel?

7. Seashell Treasures

Take a moment to appreciate the seashells scattered along the shoreline. Hold a seashell to your ear and hear not just the sound of the waves but also the whisper of the sea creatures that once called it home. Each seashell tells a unique story of the being that crafted it. Reflect on the effort and artistry involved in creating these protective shells. Consider the seashells as gifts from the ocean, a tangible reminder of the underwater world's beauty.

Hold a seashell in your hand and contemplate the intricate details, imagining the creature that once inhabited it. What challenges did it face, and what moments of beauty did it experience in the ocean? How does putting yourself in its place enhance your empathy for all living beings?

How does listening to the echo of the sea creatures' home evoke a sense of connection with the vast history of the ocean? Reflect on the shared essence of life between humans and these ancient marine inhabitants.

How does the unique design of the seashell crafted by nature inspire your appreciation for the artistic brilliance of the natural world? Reflect on the creativity inherent in every corner of the ocean, reminding us of its wonders.

8. Honoring the Ocean's Gift
Reflect on the life-giving oxygen produced by the ocean's marine life and its profound impact on all of existence. Consider how the very breaths you take are interconnected with the ocean's capacity to generate oxygen. As you breathe in, express gratitude for this vital gift and recognize the responsibility humans have in preserving the ocean's health.

How does it feel to acknowledge that the breath you just took is intimately linked to the ocean's ability to produce oxygen?

9. The Ocean's Relationship to the Climate
Reflect on the ocean's vast influence, shaping weather patterns and global temperatures. Contemplate how its currents distribute heat and moisture, regulating Earth's temperature like a natural thermostat. Acknowledge the intricate interplay between the ocean and the atmosphere, orchestrating the symphony of the Earth's climate.

How does this balance inspire a sense of awe for the precision of nature?

Close your eyes and visualize different temperature zones around the world.

Slowly move your hands through the air, sensing the imaginary temperatures changing. Feel the warmth of tropical regions and the coolness of polar areas. How do these temperature sensations within your fingertips help you embody the diverse climate patterns shaped by the ocean's influence?

Closing

In the expansive embrace of the ocean, your heart overflows with gratitude for its profound contributions to humanity and the planet. Appreciate the tranquil solace it provides, its waves whispering serenity to your soul. Thank the ocean for its life-giving essence, sustaining diverse ecosystems and providing nourishment for countless species, including humans. Express deep appreciation for its role in regulating Earth's climate, balancing temperatures, and fostering the delicate equilibrium necessary for all life to flourish. The ocean's hidden depths harbor mysteries that continue to inspire awe and wonder, reminding you of the limitless beauty of the natural world. With profound reverence, offer your gratitude for the ocean's ceaseless efforts, shaping the world in ways both seen and unseen.

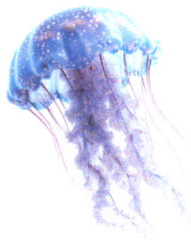

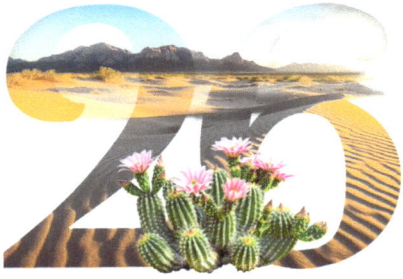

THE SERENITY OF ARID LANDS

Step into the mesmerizing desert realm, where the beauty of nature unfolds amidst unique geographical and ecological diversity. Find a quiet spot amidst the golden sands and let the desert's grace inspire your senses and offer serenity to your soul.

With every breath feel the pulse of the desert and let the land's essence merge with your very being, connecting you to its ancient soul. With each exhale, release any tension, allowing your soul to dance with the arid winds, embracing the profound serenity of this unique landscape.

1. Arrival and Grounding

Begin by standing barefoot on the warm desert sand. Feel the grains beneath your feet, connecting with the Earth's ancient wisdom. Let the desert warmth seep into your skin, embracing you with its gentle touch. Take a few deep breaths, inhaling the subtle scent of desert flora carried by the gentle breeze. Sense the vastness of the desert around you, appreciating the wide-open spaces and endless horizons.

> Sit down and touch the desert sand with your hands, feeling its texture and warmth. As you hold the sand, consider the millions of years it took to form this ancient landscape. How does the timeless nature of the desert ground you in the awareness of the passage of time, and how does it reflect the essence of your own journey?

> As you inhale the subtle scent of desert flora, how does it resonate within your body? What emotions or sensations does it evoke?

> How does the desert warmth envelop your skin? Can you feel it soothing your muscles and relaxing your body?

2. Observing Unique Features

Observe the intricate patterns formed by wind on the sand dunes and the resilient desert plants that have adapted to thrive in this arid environment. Notice how these plants conserve water and provide shelter to various desert creatures. As you gaze upon the unique geological formations, contemplate the centuries of natural artistry that have shaped the desert's rugged beauty.

> As you observe the wind-carved patterns on the sands, how does the rhythmic movement of the grains resonate with your breath and body?

> When you witness the resilient desert plants, how does their ability to thrive in challenging conditions inspire your own sense of resilience and adaptability?

> How does the wide expanse of the desert landscape make you feel?
> Can you embody the sense of vastness and freedom it offers?

3. Ecosystem Appreciation

Reflect on the significance of deserts as critical ecosystems supporting diverse forms of life. Despite their harsh conditions, deserts are home to specialized animals that have evolved remarkable adaptations. Consider the tenacity of desert life and how these species contribute to the global tapestry of biodiversity. Marvel at their ability to survive, thriving in an environment that challenges life at every turn.

> As you reflect on the significance of desert ecosystems, can you embody the tenacity and adaptability of desert animals and plants within yourself?

> How does acknowledging the diverse life forms in the desert evoke a sense of interconnectedness and unity within your own body and soul?

4. Floral Diversity

Marvel at the unique plants and cacti that thrive in these arid climates. Notice their fascinating shapes and vibrant colors, each adapted ingeniously to survive in the scarcity of water. Marvel at the persistence of these desert plants, standing firm in the rugged terrain, and allow their ability to bloom and thrive in spite of harsh conditions to fill you with awe and wonder.

> As you stand amidst desert flora, can you visualize their energy merging with your own, fostering a sense of resilience, patience, and hope within your body and soul?

How does this diversity deepen your appreciation for the complexity and beauty of life?

5. Seeds of Hope

Contemplate the silent anticipation of seeds buried in the desert sands, patiently waiting for the rains to come. Imagine the dormant life within these seeds, embodying the essence of hope and renewal. Consider the desert as a canvas where life patiently waits, reminding you of the profound cycles of nature and the resilience embedded in the tiniest of beings.

> Imagine holding a seed in your palm, feeling its weight and texture. As you breathe, visualize the potential within this tiny seed when planted in the desert soil, waiting for the rain, ready to sprout and grow. How does this imagery inspire you to consider the profound impact that a small, hopeful action can have?

> Take a moment to breathe in deeply, imagining the desert landscape transforming into a lush oasis teeming with life. As you exhale, consider the symbolic meaning of this transformation from barrenness to abundance. How does this transformation mirror your own potential for personal growth and the transformative power of hope within your soul?

6. Diverse Desert Landscapes

Acknowledge the diversity within deserts, ranging from coastal deserts kissed by the salty breath of the sea, hot and dry deserts with relentless sun, to cold deserts where snow and ice meet the arid sands, and semi-arid deserts displaying a blend of life amidst scarcity. Embrace the uniqueness of the desert you are standing in, understanding that each type offers its distinct beauty, ecosystems, and awe-inspiring landscapes.

> Find a sheltered spot in the desert, perhaps under the shade of a rare desert tree or rock formation. Feel the subtle breeze against your skin and listen to the sound of silence interrupted only by occasional whispers of the wind. How does the solitude and tranquility of the desert enhance your awareness of your own breath and presence?

> Close your eyes and visualize the diverse desert landscapes—the rolling dunes, the rocky plateaus, the sparse vegetation. As you breathe, imagine inhaling the essence of each unique desert terrain. How does the varied landscape affect your breathing and connect you to the soul of the desert?

7. Silent Guardian

Visualize the desert as a silent warrior against climate change. Acknowledge the desert's role as a carbon sink, absorbing carbon dioxide from the atmosphere and acting as a line of defense against global warming. With each breath, imagine inhaling the desert's pure, clean air, knowing that its resilience contributes to the balance of the planet's climate.

> Feel the warmth of the desert sun on your skin. How can you channel this energy to empower yourself?

> Imagine yourself as a shield against global warming, just like the desert. How can your actions and choices contribute to a cooler, more balanced world?

> As you breathe deeply, can you visualize the desert's ecosystem within your lungs, appreciating the exchange of oxygen and carbon dioxide as a vital life process?

8. Transcontinental Connection

Contemplate the fascinating connection between deserts and distant ecosystems. Ponder the Saharan sands that travel across vast oceans, carried by the wind to nourish the Amazon rainforest. Envision these tiny particles embarking on a transcontinental journey, enriching the soil of the Amazon basin and sustaining the diverse life forms of this lush jungle. Reflect on the interconnectedness of nature, where the sands of one desert nurture the vibrant life of a distant rainforest.

> Feel the desert sands beneath your feet and the rainforest's lushness in your imagination. How can you embody the harmonious balance between giving and receiving, ensuring a thriving ecosystem within your own life, relationships, and communities?

> Picture the vibrant Amazon rainforest, sustained by the desert's sands. How can you emulate this mutual support, fostering a nurturing environment where everyone's unique qualities contribute to a flourishing whole?

> How does this interconnectedness inspire a sense of global unity and the interdependence of natural systems?

Closing

Express your deepest gratitude to the desert, a realm of silent beauty that hums with the secrets of nature. The desert, a sanctuary of life, plays a crucial role in maintaining Earth's ecological harmony. Honor its awe-inspiring dance with the winds and sun, finding inspiration in its resilient soul. Carry the desert's tranquility within, a reminder of the delicate balance that sustains all living beings. Embrace the memory of its unique beauty, allowing its warmth to reside in your heart, a testament to the serene essence found in arid lands.

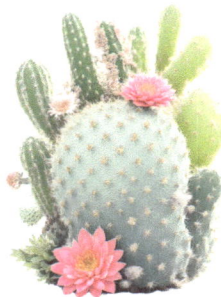

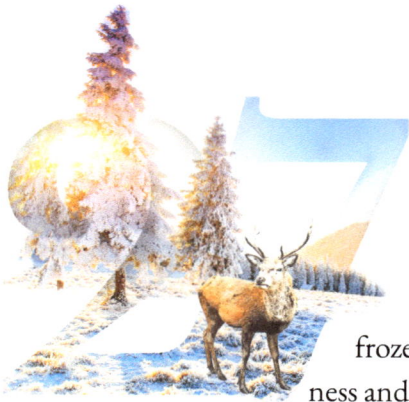

WINTER'S WHISPERS

In winter, the natural world appears to slumber beneath a pristine blanket of snow. In this serene setting, the frozen air heightens our senses, inviting us to embrace the stillness and solitude of the winter forest. As you embark on this journey, immerse yourself in the glimmering, crisp white landscape, where each tiny crystal of ice sparkles under the warm sun, illuminating the path ahead.

Begin by grounding yourself in the present moment. Take a deep breath in, allowing the cool, invigorating winter air to fill your lungs. Feel the crispness of the air energizing your body, awakening your senses. Exhale slowly, releasing any tension or stress, letting go of the outside world and surrendering to the tranquility of this winter wonderland.

1. Nature's Pristine Canvas

Contemplate the serene beauty of the snow-covered landscape, a sight that evokes a sense of purity and tranquility. Imagine each snowflake as a unique masterpiece, delicately crafted by nature's hands, collectively creating a pristine canvas beneath your feet, where the world seems to be dressed in a blanket of ethereal elegance, inviting you to step softly and cherish the artistry of the winter wonderland.

As you continue to breathe deeply, allow your awareness to expand. Notice the subtle aromas of pine and earth, carried on the chilly breeze. Feel the sensation of your breath as it mingles with the icy air, a gentle reminder of your connection to the natural world.

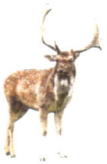

As you consider the purity of the cold air cleansing your lungs and invigorating your soul, notice the rhythm of your breathing. Are your inhalations and exhalations deeper and more intentional? How does this conscious breathing affect your sense of grounding and connection with the present moment?

2. Frozen Beauty

Take a moment to observe the intricate details of this winter wonderland. Notice how the sunlight plays upon the frozen landscape, casting a mesmerizing glow upon the snow and ice. Marvel at the beauty of nature's artwork, from the delicate frost on tree branches to the glistening icicles hanging from rocks and cliffs.

As you immerse yourself in the intricate details of this winter wonderland, how does your body respond to the beauty around you? Are there physical sensations, such as a sense of warmth or a shiver of awe, that arise as you marvel at the snowy landscape's beauty?

3. Silent masterpieces

Witness the serene beauty of the snow-covered landscape, a sight that evokes a sense of purity and tranquility. Imagine each snowflake as a unique masterpiece, collectively creating a pristine canvas beneath your feet. Reflect on the peacefulness that descends with the snow, blanketing the world in silence and inviting you to tread softly upon the Earth. Acknowledge the simplicity and elegance of this natural phenomenon, finding inspiration in its quiet magnificence.

Reflecting on the peacefulness that descends with the snow, how does your body respond to the idea of silence enveloping the world?

Are there subtle movements or shifts in your posture that reflect your inner experience of quietude?

4. Snowfall Serenity

While engaging with the snowy landscape, allow yourself to fully immerse in the peacefulness that descends with the snow, blanketing the world in silence and inviting you to embrace the profound stillness that envelops you like a soft, comforting blanket. Let the absence of sound become a canvas upon which your thoughts and emotions can gently settle, creating a tranquil sanctuary within your soul. In this hushed serenity, find solace and peace, and let the quietude of the winter landscape inspire a sense of awe and reverence for the beauty of nature's calming embrace.

As the silence of the landscape unfolds before you, how does your body resonate with the feelings of purity and tranquility that accompany this profound stillness? How does your breath change in response to this peaceful scene?

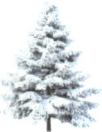

As you stand within the quietude of the landscape, consider the rhythm of your heartbeat. Does it synchronize with the calm atmosphere around you, beating in

95

harmony with the purity and tranquility of the moment? How does this awareness of your heartbeat connect you with the natural serenity of the surroundings?

5. Awakening to Winter's Embrace

Feel the brisk embrace of winter, as the air crackles with an electrifying chill that awakens every fiber of your being. Reflect on how the icy breath of the season sharpens your senses, making you acutely aware of each inhale and exhale. Consider the purity of the cold air, cleansing your lungs and invigorating your soul. Embrace the heightened awareness that comes with the frozen air, a reminder of your connection to the natural forces of nature.

How does your skin respond to the brisk embrace of winter? Are there tingling sensations or goosebumps that arise as the electrifying chill envelops you?

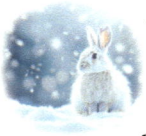

Reflecting on how the icy breath of the season sharpens your senses, observe any changes in your hearing, sight, or smell. Are you more attuned to the subtle sounds of nature, the crisp clarity of the winter landscape, or the subtle scents in the cold air? How do these heightened senses influence your overall presence and awareness?

6. Nature's Dance of Light and Ice

Visualize the gentle caress of the sun's rays, transforming the snow-covered terrain into a sparkling tapestry of shimmering crystals, each one catching the sunlight and reflecting a myriad of colors, as if the entire landscape were adorned with a thousand diamonds. Consider the interplay of light and ice, a dance that creates a mesmerizing spectacle, where every glint and glimmer becomes a testament to the harmonious collaboration between nature's elements, inviting you to witness a breathtaking masterpiece of elegance and radiance.

As you visualize the gentle caress of the sun's rays, can you feel the warmth on your skin and the subtle tingle of the sunlight? How does this imagined sensation translate into a physical response within your body, evoking a sense of comfort and connection with nature's energy?

In considering the interplay of light and ice, how do your eyes respond to the mesmerizing spectacle? Are there changes in your focus or gaze as you imagine every glint and glimmer?

Reflecting on the harmonious collaboration between nature's elements, particularly the dance of light and ice, how does your body intuitively respond to the concept of this natural partnership? Do you sense a subtle alignment or resonance within yourself, akin to the harmony witnessed in the interplay of light and ice? How does this awareness of harmony within nature influence your own sense of inner balance and equilibrium?

7. Timelessness

Ponder the concept of time in the winter forest, where the frigid temperatures suspend the flow of water, transforming it into delicate, icy sculptures that glisten in the soft sunlight like nature's own frozen masterpieces. Marvel at how this suspended animation creates a sense of timelessness, where each icicle and frost-covered branch becomes a testament to the intricate dance between nature's elements, inviting contemplation on the eternal beauty woven into the fabric of the changing seasons.

As you ponder the concept of time in the winter forest, how does your own sense of time shift? Are you aware of a slowing down or deepening of your breath, aligning with the serene pace of nature around you? How does this altered perception of time influence your awareness of the present moment?

Imagining the delicate, icy sculptures glistening in the soft sunlight, how do you envision the textures and temperatures of these frozen masterpieces? Can you feel the coolness on your skin and the smooth, icy surfaces under your fingertips? How does this sensory visualization create a tangible connection between your body and the winter landscape?

8. Tender Snowflakes

Extend your hand gently towards the snow and allow a few snowflakes to land on your skin. Notice their unique patterns and how they melt upon contact. Experience the cold, soft, and slightly wet sensation as they melt against your warmth.

As you extend your hand towards the snow, can you describe the sensation as the first snowflake makes contact with your skin? Is there a moment of coolness, followed by a gentle melting sensation? How does this tactile experience connect you with the delicate nature of each snowflake and the winter environment around you?

9. Snow's Shifting Structure

Scoop up a handful of snow and feel its varying textures. Notice how the snow feels powdery, light, and airy. Press it between your fingers, observing its malleability. Experience the sensation as it transforms from a loose powder to a compacted form in your hands.

As you scoop up a handful of snow, how does its powdery, light, and airy texture feel against your skin? Is there a sensation of coolness or weightlessness as you hold it in your hands? How does the snow's softness and lightness impact your sense of touch, inviting you to explore its delicate nature?

Fully engage your sense of touch. Press your palms gently into the snow, feeling the coolness seeping through your gloves or skin. Experience the subtle crunch as you squeeze the snow between your fingers. Pay attention to the temperature contrast between the snow and your body heat.

Pressing the snow between your fingers, can you describe the sensation of its malleability? How does the snow yield and reshape under your touch? Are there subtle shifts in its texture as you apply pressure?

How does this tactile exploration connect you with the natural resilience and adaptability of the snow, and what feelings or thoughts does it evoke?

10. Frozen Echoes

Experience the soft crunch of snow beneath your feet as you navigate the snow-covered trail, each step creating a symphony of sound that reverberates through the serene winter landscape. Take a moment to appreciate the sensory delight. With every step, you engage in a tactile dialogue with the winter ground, forging a connection that transcends words, grounding you in the present moment and peaceful rhythm of the season.

How does your body respond to the soft crunch of snow beneath your feet? Can you feel the gentle resistance and the subtle vibrations as you take each step? How does the rhythm of your walking change in response to this symphony of sounds, and how does it influence your overall sense of balance and stability?

As you appreciate the sensory delight of the snow crunching beneath your feet, are there specific sensations that stand out to you? Perhaps you notice the coldness seeping through your shoes or the way the snow molds under your weight. How do these detailed sensations contribute to your overall experience, and how do they connect you with the winter landscape in a more intimate way?

11. A Winter's Song

Listen to the melody of winter birds, their songs cutting through the crisp air, weaving a symphony that resonates with the hushed tranquility of the season. Each note, clear and crisp, carries with it the resilience of these avian creatures, their melodies echoing through the stillness and reminding us of the beauty that endures even in the chilliest of times.

> As you listen to the melody of winter birds, how does your body respond to the clear and crisp notes cutting through the crisp air? Are there physical sensations that arise, such as a tingling in your ears or a subtle shift in your posture?

> As you contemplate the endurance of beauty in the chilliest of times, how does your body respond to the reminder of resilience in the winter birds' songs? Are there feelings of inspiration or awe that manifest physically, such as a warm sensation in your chest or a softening in your muscles? How does this awareness of enduring beauty influence your own sense of strength and grace, connecting you with the innate resilience within yourself?

12. The Sun's Return

Contemplate the symbolism of the sun's return after a prolonged winter night, a metaphor for hope and renewal. As the first rays of sunlight pierce the darkness, they illuminate the world, dispelling the shadows of the night and casting a warm, golden glow upon the Earth.

> Reflecting on the dispelling of shadows and the illumination of the world, how does your posture change as you envision the arrival of sunlight? Do you find yourself standing taller or sitting more upright, embracing the metaphorical light? How does this embodiment of openness and receptivity to light and warmth reflect your own capacity for hope and renewal, and how does it influence your sense of optimism and resilience?

13. The Dormant Forest

Observe the dormant state of the winter forest, where life appears to retreat, conserving energy for the eventual rebirth of spring. Amidst the seemingly lifeless trees and hibernating animals, there is a quiet energy pulsating beneath the surface, a silent preparation for the vibrant resurgence that accompanies the arrival of spring.

As you observe the dormant state of the winter forest, can you sense a stillness settling within your own body? Are there physical sensations, like a calming of your breath or a softening of your muscles, that reflect the tranquility of the forest? How does this shared stillness deepen your connection with the natural world and bring a sense of quiet energy to your own being?

Reflecting on the forest's preparation for the vibrant resurgence of spring, how does your posture change as you envision this silent energy? Do you notice a subtle shift in your body's readiness or openness, as if you are also preparing for a new beginning? How does this embodiment of quiet energy inspire your own sense of patience and trust in the natural cycles of life, grounding you in the present moment and nurturing your anticipation for the future?

14. Ethereal Resilience

Gaze upon the skeletal branches of bare trees and bushes, stripped of their foliage. Allow your eyes to trace the intricate patterns etched against the winter sky. In this stark simplicity lies a profound elegance, inviting you to contemplate the raw beauty of their naked form. Absent leaves, these branches stand as resilient guardians, shaped by the shifting seasons, unveiling their core strength even amidst vulnerability.

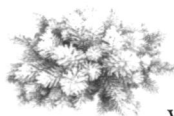

Allowing your eyes to trace the intricate patterns against the winter sky, do you find your breath naturally deepening or slowing down? How does this intentional observation influence the rhythm of your breathing, connecting you with the quiet elegance of nature's design? How does this embodiment of stillness deepen your appreciation for the winter landscape and evoke a sense of peace within your being?

Reflecting on the profound elegance found in the stark simplicity of the bare branches, how does your body respond to the invitation to contemplate their raw beauty? Can you feel a sense of awe or reverence in your physical posture, as if you are in the presence of a profound revelation?

15. In the Balance of Light and Shadow

Notice the shadows cast by winter's soft light, creating contrasts and depth in the snowy landscape, where each tree, rock, and snowdrift becomes a canvas for nature's intricate play of darkness and illumination. As the soft sunlight filters through the bare branches, the landscape transforms into a study of contrasts, with patches of warmth juxtaposed against the cool shadows. Notice the balance that exists within these contrasts, finding harmony in the acceptance of both shadow and light, recognizing that it is this delicate equilibrium that enhances the visual poetry of winter.

> Reflecting on the delicate equilibrium between shadow and light, how does your body respond to the acceptance of both aspects? Can you feel a sense of harmony or balance within yourself, mirroring the equilibrium found in the winter scene?

> How does this awareness of balance enhance your connection with the visual poetry of winter, fostering a deeper appreciation for the interplay of shadows and light in the natural world and within your own being?

16. Unveiled

Observe or imagine the wildlife moving amidst the winter landscape, unobstructed by the dense foliage of warmer seasons. With the absence of leaves, the once-hidden creatures now traverse the snowcovered ground with a sense of purpose, their movements unmasked and unfiltered. Reflect on the transparency and visibility that winter brings, allowing you to witness the natural world with clarity, where every darting rabbit, graceful deer, and soaring bird becomes a visible testament to the intricate web of life. In this open expanse, the winter landscape offers a rare opportunity for unhindered observation, inviting you to marvel at the fluidity of the animal kingdom, appreciating the seamless interactions that unfold before your eyes.

> Considering every animal as a visible testament to the intricate web of life, how does your awareness of their presence impact your own sense of belonging within this ecosystem?

> Can you feel a sense of humility and interconnectedness as you witness these creatures navigating the winter landscape?

> How does this awareness of the interdependence of all living beings enhance your own embodiment, grounding you in the present moment and fostering a deeper understanding of the harmonious relationships within nature?

17. Snow and Moonlight

Notice or imagine the transformative power of snow, turning the darkest night into a softly illuminated wonderland where each snowflake reflects the moonlight like a tiny, glimmering gem. As the snow falls gently from the sky, it blankets the world in a pristine, ethereal glow, casting a serene ambiance that defies the darkness. In this transformation, even the harshest winter night is softened, and the world seems to hold its breath, captivated by the mesmerizing interplay of snow and moonlight.

> Imagining the snow falling gently from the sky, how does your body respond to the imagery of the world being blanketed in a pristine, ethereal glow? Are there moments of stillness or expansiveness within your own being, mirroring the serene ambiance of the snow-covered landscape?

> How does this sensory experience of snow and moonlight invite you to cultivate a sense of inner peace and quietude, grounding you in the present moment?

> Can you sense a shared sense of awe and wonder within your own being, aligning with the harmony of nature's elements? How does this embodiment of awe and reverence deepen your connection with the natural world, inspiring a sense of reverence for the transformative power of the winter night, and how does it evoke a sense of gratitude within you for the beauty that surrounds you?

18. Hibernation's Healing Silence

Consider the wisdom of hibernation, a time for trees, plants, and animals to rest and recuperate, embracing the essential cycle of renewal in the natural world. As the cold embrace of winter settles in, these living beings retreat into a state of dormancy, conserving their energy and resources. It's a period of profound stillness, where growth takes place beneath the surface, roots draw nourishment from the earth, and animals find sanctuary in their burrows.

> Reflecting on the wisdom of hibernation, how does your body respond to the idea of embracing a state of rest and recuperation? Can you feel a sense of relaxation or release in your muscles, as if your body is acknowledging the importance of rejuvenation?

> Within nature's intentional pause, reflect on the balance between activity and rest, appreciating the necessity of both in your journey toward mindfulness, self-discovery, and growth.

Closing

In the hush of winter, offer gratitude for the moments of calm introspection, the glistening wonder of snowflakes adorning the Earth, and the profound lessons of resilience discovered in nature's quiet slumber. Express thanks for the tranquility that allowed you to delve deep within yourself and for the gentle transformation that winter's touch bestowed upon you. Carry a heart full of gratitude, appreciating the subtle beauty found in the stillness, the promise of renewal, and the knowledge that winter's wisdom will accompany you on your journey into the blooming embrace of spring.

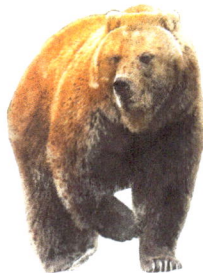

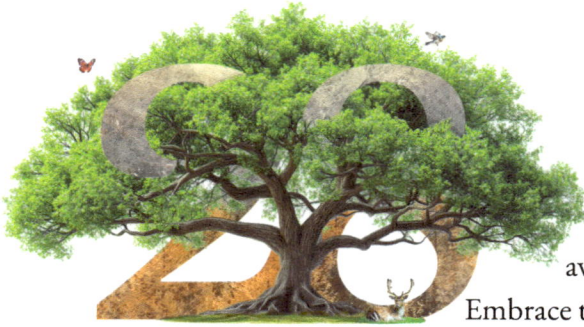

SACRED CONVERSATIONS

Find a quiet spot in the heart of the forest, away from the hustle and bustle of everyday life. Embrace the tranquility around you and let the natural world envelop your senses. Today, embark on a unique nature-based therapy experience by engaging in a conversation with a wise and ancient tree. Trees, with their centuries of existence, are patient listeners, nonjudgmental beings, and masters of the art of holding your words in utmost privacy. They stand tall, their branches reaching out like open arms, ready to embrace your thoughts and emotions in a sanctuary of trust and understanding.

1. Find Your Tree
Pause for a moment and take a deep, cleansing breath, filling your lungs with the pure essence of the forest. Inhale slowly, allowing the crisp, rejuvenating air to energize your body and clear your mind. As you exhale, release any tension, letting go of the outside world. Feel yourself becoming one with the natural surroundings. With each breath, let the forest's tranquility seep into your being. Stroll among the trees, tuning in to the subtle whispers of the leaves and the earthy fragrance that surrounds you. Wait until you feel a gentle pull, a silent invitation from one particular tree. Trust your instincts—it is nature guiding you to your silent, patient listener.

2. Introduce Yourself
Approach the tree with respect. Gently place your hand on its bark, feeling the rough textures beneath your fingertips. Close your eyes, take a deep breath, and introduce yourself silently, using your thoughts. Feel the tree's energy, and let it acknowledge your presence.

3. Ask Your Life Question
With your hand still resting on the tree, ask it a question that weighs on your mind. It could be about your life's purpose, a difficult decision, or simply seeking guidance. Imagine the question flowing from your heart to the tree, like a whispered secret.

4. Share Something Private
Open your heart to the tree. Share something private, something you've never told anyone

else. Trust the ancient wisdom of the tree to hold your words sacred. Feel the release as your secrets are absorbed into the tree's essence, leaving you feeling lighter.

5. Share Your Sorrow

Acknowledge any sorrow or pain you carry within you. Express your feelings to the tree, allowing the natural environment to bear witness to your emotions. Let the tree absorb your sorrow, offering you solace in return.

6. Ask for Advice

Finally, ask the tree for advice. Imagine its roots reaching deep into the Earth, drawing upon ancient wisdom. Listen with your heart, not just your ears. The tree might respond in the rustling of leaves or the creaking of branches. Be open to the subtle messages nature imparts.

Closing

With gratitude in your heart, gently withdraw your hand from the tree, feeling the lingering warmth of its energy. As you step away, carry the tree's wisdom, the shared secrets, and the comforting embrace of the forest with you. Remember, whenever life's questions weigh heavily on your soul, you can return to this sacred space, where ancient trees stand as guardians of your deepest thoughts and emotions. The forest will always be there, patiently waiting, ready to welcome you back into its tranquil arms.

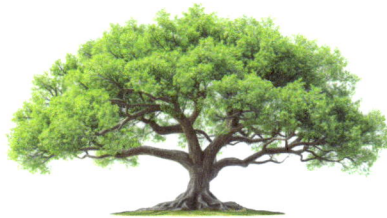

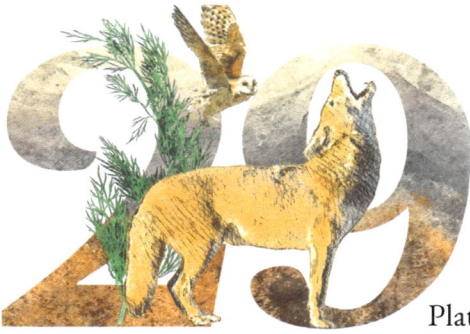

EXPLORING THE INVISIBLE SOUL WITHIN NATURE

The world of soul is invisible. The Greek philosopher, Plato, was the first to describe the world as a living thing, "truly endowed with soul and intelligence."[16] In our daily life, we often talk about things with utmost certainty. Yet, our universe extends beyond what we can perceive with our senses. Its mysterious, underlying reality is often hidden from us, yet its unseen existence is essential for giving rise to things that we sense. The hidden is as real as the visible.

The silence of time, consciousness, thoughts, imagination, and air were at one time mystifying. Each of them keeping to itself, each of them challenging our commonsense notion of what we see. We are limited beings participating in a world where nature is busy at work beneath the surface, where we encounter the generosity of invisible elements ruled by invisible truths. We live between the known and unknown. Between the visible and invisible. Between the revealed and unrevealed. Between darkness and light.

Beyond the realm of visibility, the soul embodies the deepest essence, an underlying presence that provides all things with an internal dimension. Regardless of its outward appearance or the complexity of the system, every entity harbors a concealed inner universe.

Find a serene spot in the heart of the forest. Sit or stand comfortably, grounding yourself in the natural surroundings. Close your eyes gently and take a few deep breaths. As you breathe in, imagine you are inhaling the essence of the forest, and as you exhale, release any tension or thoughts that may weigh you down. Allow yourself to enter a state of calm and receptivity.

1. Acknowledging the Invisible Soul

With your eyes closed, visualize the invisible soul within the forest. Imagine it as a vibrant, glowing energy that interweaves with the trees, the soil, and the very air you breathe. Feel its presence around you, holding you in a warm, gentle embrace.

---

16   Jowett, Benjamin. "Timaeus by Plato," The Internet Classics Archive, https://classics.mit.edu/Plato/timaeus.html. Accessed on July 13, 2024.

How does it feel to connect with the invisible soul within nature? How did the visualization of the invisible soul within nature make you feel? Were there specific emotions or sensations that arose during this visualization?

2. Connecting with the Unseen Energy

Extend your senses beyond the visible and tangible. Feel the subtle energy of the trees, the rustle of leaves, and the whispers of the wind. Sense how the invisible soul of nature communicates with you through these subtle cues. Allow yourself to be enveloped by this energy.

What subtle cues or sensations did you notice while connecting with the unseen energy?

Did you experience a sense of peace or harmony?

3. Reflecting on the Invisible Bond

Contemplate the subtle energy exchanges that occur, allowing it to reshape your perception of the forest. Allow yourself to marvel at the intricate harmony that exists between you and the trees, recognizing the shared life force that pulses through both your veins and the natural world, weaving you seamlessly into the tapestry of all existence.

Reflect on how this connection makes you perceive the forest in a new light.

How has your perception of the forest changed after acknowledging the invisible soul within it? Did you experience a deeper sense of belonging?

4. Exploring Inner Stillness

In the presence of the invisible soul within nature, embrace inner stillness. Listen to the silence between the sounds of the forest. Observe how this stillness allows you to delve deeper into your own thoughts and feelings.

How does the soul of the world see and sense you?

What emotions, sensations, or wonderings emerged during the moments of inner stillness?

How did the moments of inner stillness deepen your connection with your inner self?

5. Embracing the Unseen

In the embrace of nature's serenity, take a moment to delve deeply into the essence of the invisible soul that resides within every leaf, every creature, and every whisper of the wind. Reflect upon the profound significance of this unseen force, the essence that connects all living things in a harmonious dance of existence.

Imagine the intricate web of connections that extend beyond the visible world—the subtle energy that courses through the veins of ancient trees, the silent communication among wildlife, and the unseen bonds that unite the entire ecosystem. Picture the delicate balance maintained by this invisible soul, nurturing life in its many forms and sustaining the natural world. With each breath, let the awareness of this invisible soul settle within you, filling your heart with a sense of wonder and reverence. Recognize that you, too, are a part of this intricate tapestry, intertwined with the soul of nature.

How has your perspective on nature shifted after acknowledging the presence of the invisible soul within it? Did you gain a sense of interconnectedness with the environment?

Closing

In the quiet embrace of nature, express your deepest gratitude for the unseen forces that shape the world, embracing the timeless presence of the invisible soul within nature. Acknowledge the unseen threads that weave us all together, connecting every living being and every moment in time. Its wisdom whispers through the wind, its strength echoes in the mountains, and its gentleness flows in the rivers. Its eternal presence reminds us of the beauty in every breath, the unity in every heartbeat, and the love in every shared experience. With profound appreciation, honor the soul of the world's boundless existence, embracing the infinite tapestry of life that the world's soul so beautifully creates.

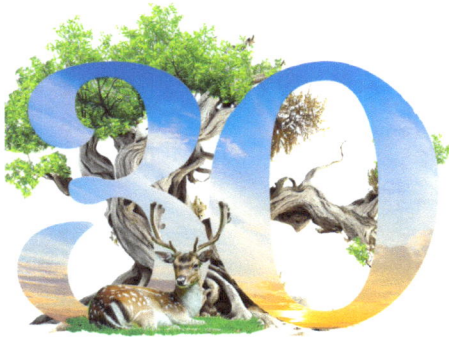

END OF DAY
CLOSING MEDITATIONS

Meditation 1

Form a circle. Take three slow, deep breaths. Inhale deeply, inviting the essence of life to fill your being; exhale, surrendering to its infinite wisdom.

As our nature-based therapy journey comes to an end, let us express gratitude for the deep attention and playful spirit that accompanied us today. With each rustle of leaves, every birdsong, and the soft caress of the wind, we have immersed ourselves in the wonders of nature, learning to observe with more profound awareness and embracing the playful curiosity within us. Embrace the possibility that you are intricately interwoven into an endlessly evolving, vibrant relationship with every entity you encounter. Invite your heart to be receptive to the understanding that despite our differences, a unifying thread weaves through all beings.

Take a moment to acknowledge the newfound relationships you've nurtured—with the natural world and within yourself. Feel the grounding energy of the Earth beneath your feet and the wisdom of ancient trees whispering their secrets in the wind. As you stand here, remember that this experience isn't confined to this moment; it lingers within you, shaping your perception and understanding of the world.

With hearts full of gratitude, let us carry this sense of deep attention and playfulness into our daily lives. Whether amidst the bustling city streets or the quietude of our homes, may we continue to observe the world with fresh eyes and approach each moment with the playful curiosity of a child.

Thank you, nature, for being our guide and companion on this enriching journey. As we depart, we do so with a renewed soul and a deeper understanding of the intricate dance between humanity and the natural world. Until we meet again, may your days be filled with the gentle embrace of nature's wisdom and the playful curiosity that keeps our hearts forever young.

Exercise:
Close your eyes, grounding yourself in the present moment. Feel the Earth beneath you, supporting your every breath and intention. Inhale deeply, inviting nature's energy into your being; exhale, surrendering to the interconnectedness of all things and finding harmony within.

1. Wish for the Earth
In the sanctuary of your heart, visualize our beautiful planet, teeming with life and the breathtaking wonders of nature. As you inhale, nurture a sincere wish within your heart for the Earth, envisioning a tomorrow where it thrives, where ecosystems flourish, and where peace reigns supreme. As you exhale, imagine your wish radiating outward, blending seamlessly with the soul of the world.

2. Wish for the Person on Your Right:
Now, turn your focus to the person on your right, whether physically present or in your thoughts. Reflect on their journey, their dreams, and their struggles. As you inhale, channel your empathy into a heartfelt wish for their wellbeing. As you exhale, envision your heartfelt wish extending towards the person beside you, enveloping them in a warm embrace.

3. Wish for Yourself
Lastly, turn your attention inward. Acknowledge your own aspirations, dreams, and the love you deserve. In this moment, make a wish for yourself. As you inhale, visualize your mind immersed in stillness and your heart embraced by peace. With each exhalation, visualize your heartfelt wish sailing into the cosmos, blending seamlessly with the soul of the world and the profound depths of your own heart.

With these wishes, open your eyes, carrying the positive energy you've cultivated today into the world, nurturing kindness and understanding within yourself and of others.

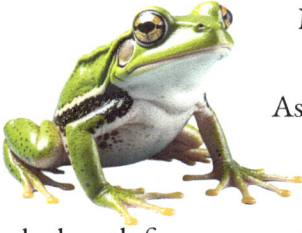

Meditation 2

As we come to the end of this rejuvenating day, let's take a moment to ground ourselves in gratitude and serenity. Close your eyes gently and inhale deeply, feeling the crisp forest air fill your lungs. Hold the breath for a moment, embracing the essence of the ancient trees surrounding us. Now, exhale slowly, releasing any tension or worries, allowing them to dissolve into the earth beneath.

In this tranquil moment, sense the interconnectedness of all living things, feeling the rhythm of nature harmonize with your own heartbeat. In closing, let us extend our heartfelt gratitude to all the kindred souls drawn to the natural world, each one forging a profound and conscious connection with nature. Your presence, like a gentle breeze through the leaves, enriches the collective experience, reminding us of the intricate threads that bind us to the natural world.

Together, we embark on a journey of mindful exploration, honoring the sanctity of nature and nurturing a deeper, more conscious relationship with our Earth. Your emotional resonance with the natural world illuminates the path for others, weaving a tapestry of awareness and reverence that stretches far beyond these moments.

With gratitude, we celebrate the shared commitment to preserve, protect, and cherish the wonders of our earthly home.

Exercise

Close your eyes, grounding yourself in the present moment. Feel the Earth beneath you, supporting your every breath and intention. Inhale deeply, inviting nature's energy into your being; exhale, surrendering to the interconnectedness of all things and finding harmony within.

1. Wish for the Earth

In the sanctuary of your heart, visualize our beautiful planet, teeming with life and the breathtaking wonders of nature. As you inhale, nurture a sincere wish within your heart for the Earth, envisioning a tomorrow where it thrives, where ecosystems flourish, and where peace reigns supreme. As you exhale, imagine your wish radiating outward, blending seamlessly with the soul of the world.

2. Wish for the Person on Your Right

Now, turn your focus to the person on your right, whether physically present or in your thoughts. Reflect on their journey, their dreams, and their struggles. As you inhale, channel your empathy into a heartfelt wish for their wellbeing. As you exhale, envision your heartfelt wish extending towards the person beside you, enveloping them in a warm embrace.

3. Wish for Yourself

Lastly, turn your attention inward. Acknowledge your own aspirations, dreams, and the love you deserve. In this moment, make a wish for yourself. As you inhale, visualize your mind immersed in stillness and your heart embraced by peace. As you exhale, visualize your heartfelt wish sailing into the cosmos, blending seamlessly with the soul of the world and the profound depths of your own heart.

With these wishes, open your eyes, carry this peace and the positive energy you've cultivated today into the world, nurturing kindness, understanding, and deepening connections.

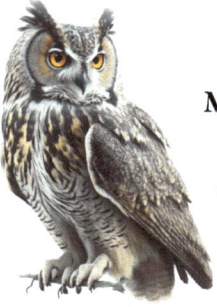

Meditation 3

Close your eyes, grounding yourself in the present moment. Feel the Earth beneath you, supporting your every breath and intention. Breathe in the rich aroma of damp earth and ancient pines. Hold your breath, allowing yourself to become fully immersed in the essence of all life that surrounds you. In this moment of profound stillness, consciously invite nature's energy into your being.

Within the forest's embrace, let a profound sense of gratitude for nature swell within your heart. Acknowledge the profound interconnectivity, unparalleled beauty, and life-giving essence that weave through every aspect of the natural world. With each breath, you become a part of the intricate tapestry, interwoven with the threads that bind all living things, resonating with the harmonious pulse of existence.

In closing, extend your deepest gratitude to the Earth. As you immerse yourself in the beauty and intricacies of nature, let this experience kindle a profound commitment to care for and protect this precious planet. Embrace the responsibility to preserve the delicate balance of our environment, ensuring the continued harmony of the natural world for generations to come.

Exercise

Close your eyes, grounding yourself in the present moment. Feel the Earth beneath you, supporting your every breath and intention. Inhale deeply, inviting nature's energy into your being; exhale, surrendering to the interconnectedness of all things and finding harmony within.

1. Wish for the Earth

In the sanctuary of your heart, visualize our beautiful planet, teeming with life and the breathtaking wonders of nature. As you inhale, nurture a sincere wish within your heart for the Earth, envisioning a tomorrow where it thrives, where ecosystems flourish, and where peace reigns supreme. As you exhale, imagine your wish radiating outward, blending seamlessly with the soul of the world.

2. Wish for the Person on Your Right

Now, turn your focus to the person on your right, whether physically present or in your thoughts. Reflect on their journey, their dreams, and their struggles. As you inhale, channel your empathy into a heartfelt wish for their wellbeing. As you exhale, envision your heartfelt wish extending towards the person beside you, enveloping them in a warm embrace.

3. Wish for Yourself

Lastly, turn your attention inward. Acknowledge your own aspirations, dreams, and the love you deserve. In this moment, make a wish for yourself. As you inhale, visualize your mind immersed in stillness and your heart embraced by peace. As you exhale, visualize your heartfelt wish sailing into the cosmos, blending seamlessly with the soul of the world and the profound depths of your own heart.

With these wishes, open your eyes, carry this peace and the positive energy you've cultivated today into the world, nurturing kindness, understanding, and deepening connections.

Crossing into a forest is not just a step on a trail,
but a deliberate movement into a space where you co-mingle
in a timeless union with the sacred.

Appendix for Group Facilitators: Rules for a Safe, Creative, and Collaborative Group Environment

Have you ever started to listen to someone speak and thought, "Yeah, I already know that," or, "I doubt that's true," or, "Wow, are they ever disconnected from reality!"?

We often don't give much thought to all the beliefs and assumptions that are structuring the ways we see the world. Fixed ideas paralyze our abilities to change, adapt, and appreciate an-other's view. Whether consciously or unconsciously, we tend to live our lives with a list of 'certainties' or assumptions. We are inclined to interpret information with a tendency toward reinforcing preexisting convictions. We cannot listen in a way to fully understand an-other if we have locked down our minds with our own point of view. This way of participating in life is limiting. When we suspend the beliefs, opinions, and judgments that we subscribe to, we suspend our egos, allowing possibilities for new relationships and new understandings between different perspectives to take place.

In discussions, people may choose to share a personal response or thought. Your response must be supportive, open, and lead with a "Yes, and. . ." approach. Saying "yes" isn't always about agreeing with someone. It is about affirming their feelings or thoughts. The "and" allows you to add to the conversation with your ideas. This technique moves the conversation forward, increases interaction, encourages everyone to fully participate, and allows everyone to experience the most out of the conversation.

IDA M. COVI—BIO

Ida Covi is an eco-psychologist with a graduate degree in depth psychology. She serves as the CEO of the international think tank, iRewild Institute. Ida has received recognition for her outstanding work, including Pacifica Graduate Institute's highest award, the Chancellor's Award for Excellence. She is the author of the books "Rewilding The Senses," "Even The Caterpillar Sings," and "ReachingBeyond," along with many professional articles.

Growing up on a farm, Ida developed a profound bond with the natural world as she dwelt amidst the presence of countless animals. It's where she first learned that all beings cherish their lives and share the same desire to live as we do. It served as a reminder of the inherent intelligence, preciousness, and irreplaceability of every single being. From then on, she relished in the scent of pine forests, the tender breath of her horse, the solace of starry nights, and the unforgettable adventures exploring nature's hidden corners while experiencing its deepest mysteries.

iREWILD INSTITUTE

iRewild.com
iRewild Institute is an international think tank of transdisciplinary thought leaders committed to helping people forge a deeper, more conscious relationship with nature as we work toward creating a world in which we all belong.

iRewild Institute envisions a world where ecological consciousness is not just an idea, but a deeply ingrained way of life for every individual and community. We strive to lead a global movement that fundamentally transforms how humanity perceives and interacts with the natural world, ensuring that every decision we make contributes to the restoration and flourishing of our planet's ecosystems. By uniting the collective wisdom of diverse thought leaders and collaborating with organizations, entrepreneurs, researchers, and communities, we aim to inspire and implement innovative solutions that drive meaningful and lasting change. Our vision is to create a world where all beings are valued, where every life form thrives, and where humanity works in harmony with nature to secure a sustainable future for all life on Earth.

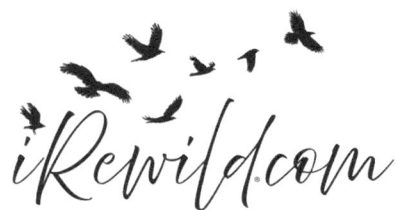

www.ingramcontent.com/pod-product-compliance
Lightning Source LLC
Chambersburg PA
CBHW060811270326
41928CB00003B/52